Science of Successful Supervision and Mentorship

Science of Successful Supervision and Mentorship

Linda S. Carozza

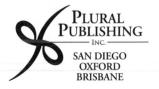

PLURAL
PUBLISHING
INC.

SAN DIEGO
OXFORD
BRISBANE

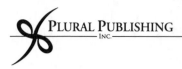

5521 Ruffin Road
San Diego, CA 92123

e-mail: info@pluralpublishing.com
Web site: http://www.pluralpublishing.com

49 Bath Street
Abingdon, Oxfordshire OX14 1EA
United Kingdom

FSC
Mixed Sources
Product group from well-managed
forests and other controlled sources

Cert no. SW-COC-002283
www.fsc.org
© 1996 Forest Stewardship Council

Copyright © by Plural Publishing, Inc. 2011

Typeset in 11/14 Garamond book by Flanagan's Publishing Services, Inc.
Printed in the United States of America by McNaughton & Gunn

ISBN-13: 978-1-59756-184-6
ISBN-10: 1-59756-184-3

Library of Congress Cataloging-in-Publication Data

Carozza, Linda S.
  Science of successful supervision and mentorship / Linda S. Carozza.
       p. ; cm.
  Includes bibliographical references and index.
  ISBN-13: 978-1-59756-184-6 (alk. paper)
  ISBN-10: 1-59756-184-3 (alk. paper)
  1. Medical students—Supervision of. 2. Mentoring in medicine.
  3. Mentoring in medicine—Case studies. I. Title.
  [DNLM: 1. Speech-Language Pathology—organization & administration.
  2. Mentors. WL 340.2]
  R737.C37 2010
  610.71—dc22

                                                                    2010042140

Contents

Appendixes

Foreword

Successful supervision and mentoring require a unique blending of both art and science. As a science, supervision incorporates principles of evidence-based practice, professional standards, and ethical practice. In its art form, successful supervision and mentoring require the knowledge and skills to solve problems, promote creativity, manage diversity, and manage conflict.

Dr. Linda Carozza's *Science of Successful Supervision and Mentorship* offers the clinician a new and updated look at this unique blending of art and science to promote effective supervision and mentoring. Practitioners with experience and those new to their roles as supervisors and mentors will benefit from the overview of history in supervision research and current trends in models of supervision included in this book.

The author provides an in-depth discussion of the differences between mentoring and supervision, reflective practice (self supervision), multicultural issues, professional ethics, and the need for evidence-based practice with application to supervision. By providing case studies and reflective exercises, the reader is able to fully explore competencies and strategies for effective supervision and mentoring in any clinical setting.

Throughout this remarkable book, Dr. Carozza provides the reader with excellent references, citing the works of key contributors to the area of supervision and mentoring. *Science of Successful Supervision and Mentorship* should be a primary resource for anyone engaged in this most important aspect of the profession.

Melanie W. Hudson, MA, CCC-SLP

Preface

In my career I have had amazing experiences I could have never anticipated as a young woman: I have seen people talk for the first time after a stroke. I have seen people discard feeding tubes and eat again. I have been there when babies uttered their first words to their parents, and many other first-time teachable moments. I learned far more from the families than I ever taught them. This awakening inspired me to tell my clinical story, to explore the art as well as the science of my chosen profession, to practice, teach, and mentor. It is my sincere hope that by introducing the concepts contained in this book, individuals who follow in the profession will be graced with the rewarding experience of a lifetime of service that I enjoy.

This book is the collaborative work of a career that spans more than 35 years as a certified speech-language pathologist and clinical supervisor with clinical experience in a variety of different settings. I have worked closely with students for most of my career and have witnessed first hand some of the unique challenges that arise as a result of being a supervisor. My particular interest lies in working with students of diverse backgrounds and I strongly feel that there is a great need for supervision and mentorship of multicultural students. Issues of cultural diversity that hold particular influence on the supervisory process in speech-language pathology are detailed throughout the book. My purpose in writing this book is for it to serve as a resource guide for professionals in the field of speech-language pathology, as well as a compilation of the development of the processes, parameters, and approaches to supervision in the field of speech-language pathology.

This book was written by a clinical practitioner with practitioners and real-world contexts in mind. It may be used with other supervision texts, by itself, or in workshops and training seminars. It contains real-life examples of clinical case scenarios, supervisory dialogues and reflections, as well as personal accounts of mentorship and supervisory experiences. It also looks at supervision from multiple perspectives—including special attention to bilingual/multicultural populations. Some individuals may find that the material will help them make sense and meaning of the theories and research, whereas others will want to focus on the literature review to develop the necessary background knowledge. How you read and use this book depends on your own preference and learning style.

Focus

This book is not a "how-to" book, but rather a "here's how" book. It is meant to serve as a resource guide for professionals to develop a better understanding of the supervisory process, a topic that frequently is not covered at the undergraduate or graduate level coursework.

This book focuses on the current challenges in the field of speech-language pathology and the research available to meet those needs. Secondarily, the book addresses the issue of mentorship and how sound practice of mentorship principles can relate to a satisfying and fulfilling career. The introductory section describes the early history of speech-language pathology supervision research. Second, the scientific underpinnings of successful supervision are reviewed, along with the competencies a successful supervisor should seek to attain according to research, anecdotal evidence, and practice standards. Last, supportive contexts for supervision and mentorship are explored.

The concept of supervision and mentorship at various career stages is also explored, with undergraduate training differentiated from graduate and postgraduate education. This book is a combination of both factual and experiential information, which is reflected in the various types of content and writing styles presented.

Chapter Highlights

Chapter 1 provides the reader with a general overview of the basic principles of supervision and mentorship, including important concepts and definitions of the terms used throughout this book. It also looks at some of the relevant history of research in supervision, beginning with the earlier models and continuing into current models. Chapter 2 addresses some of the current issues in supervision research. Chapter 3 examines some novel approaches to addressing these issues using current research. Some of the variables influencing the supervisor-supervisee relationship are discussed and illustrated using case study examples. Chapter 4 continues the discussion of some of the issues inherent in clinical supervision as well as some expert opinions relating to supervision and mentorship. Included are key elements for developing self-awareness through metacognitive activities. Chapter 5 examines issues of accountability in supervision and mentorship and includes an in-depth discussion related to the ASHA Code of Ethics and how this guides our clinical practice. Chapter 6 highlights several important competencies which supervisors should possess. It also explores several strategies based on current research trends (i.e., conversational analysis, reflective practice, personal narratives) that may be useful to incorporate into one's clinical practice.

Chapter 7 examines an area currently at the forefront of the speech-language pathology discipline—evidence-based practice. Chapter 8 delves into a thorough explanation of mentorship and supervision. Chapter 9, written by Andrea Moxley, Associate Director of ASHA's Multicultural Resources, provides a valuable contribution to this book by describing the ASHA S.T.E.P. mentoring program. Chapter 10, written by Patrick Walden, Associate Professor at St. John's University, looks at some future directions for clinical supervision. Finally, Chapter 11 gives an overview of all of the important issues and concepts presented throughout this book.

Reflections on Supervisory Goals and Objectives

In general, it is simpler to describe concepts such as what supervision seeks to accomplish as opposed to how the process can be accomplished and replicated, as the professional and psychosocial relationship is reciprocal and affected by a myriad of variables. It is a learning process for both students and supervisors, which promotes both personal and professional growth. Excellent supervisors seek to become exemplary and to act as a guide and a role model for their students. Alternatively, students look to their supervisors for the necessary guidance and support to steer them on their journey. Although the majority of clinicians report positive clinical fellowship year experiences, the difficulties that may arise likely are complex and require an understanding of both clinical and ethical practice in the discipline.

We are frequently assigned the role of supervisor without fully understanding everything that that role entails, and having only our own personal experiences to go by. This can be problematic in that the development of good supervisory skills can take many years, and requires a very different skill set than that to which we are accustomed. In this respect, this book is meant to help professionals broaden their scope of thinking by considering principles relevant to supervision including self-reflection, self-analysis, and self-monitoring. It is important to keep in mind that good clinical skills require a metacognitive awareness of oneself and others.

It is clear that supervision and mentorship requirements are different for undergraduates, graduates, and working professionals. However, the book is geared toward supervision and mentorship as general constructs. It is intended for use by professionals in the field of speech-language pathology at all levels, both those who have just embarked on their career paths as well as seasoned supervisors and clinicians. It is based on the collective wisdom of many sources, encompassing both academic rigor and personal experiences of studying and practicing in the field of speech-language pathology. The general principles of communication and leadership from allied professions are explored. The theoretical perspective taken by this book is interdisciplinary in nature and, although I do not go into the theories in detail (other books do that), we apply the theories to the supervision process. Aspects of learning styles, psychology of the self as well as others, and even business practices are incorporated.

This book addresses recent thinking in the areas of supervisor accountability and objective measures of supervision vis à vis data collection. This is an area of study that goes back several decades.

According to Oratio (1977), supervisory objectives include many key variables. Oratio (1977) cited the understanding and utilization of human dynamics, establishing clear objectives, observation, and analysis of the "teaching-learning act": providing feedback, knowledge of theory, materials, practice, and research, maintenance of objectivity, challenging and motivating student clinicians, and appreciation of individual differences. Furthermore, Oratio (1977) stated that the two primary operational objectives of clinical supervision are: (1) to affect a change in clinician behavior that will in turn modify client learning positively, and (2) to encourage growth and independence of students to independent clinicians. In this very insightful work, the author describes many of the current dynamics that are critical in current models, such as the use of illustrative training scenarios and self-reflection.

The requisite communication skills of a supervisor are also detailed, along with many of the most relevant topics in supervision from standards to challenging case studies, from the standpoint of the American Speech-Language-Hearing Association (ASHA), as well as researchers from allied areas. In my own practice, I have witnessed that supervision has evolved along with changing cultural patterns in our increasingly diverse society. Therefore, cultural issues surrounding supervision are examined extensively. This is especially relevant in today's institutions of higher education with many students of diverse backgrounds.

Another form of supervision may take place when speech-language pathologists supervise support personnel. This is the case in certain states in which there is a licensed designation for speech-language pathology assistants. The ASHA Task Force on Support Personnel (1996) has developed a guidelines and training document titled "Guidelines for the Training, Use, and Supervision of Speech-Language Pathology Assistants." However, this is a specialized interest area that goes beyond the intended scope of this book.

The American Speech-Language-Hearing Association (2007a) has issued a position paper on the responsibilities of individuals who mentor clinical fellows as an Issues in Ethics Statement, presented in the Appendix of this text. This underscores that ASHA sees the clinical fellowship year as the intersection between mentorship and supervision. This distinction is further explored in later chapters. First, the current research detailed in this book aims to delineate objective measures of superior supervision in an effort to provide standards of evidence-based practice. It is important to note that whereas this book attempts to examine the scientific under-pinnings of supervision, there currently exists more qualitative rather than quantitative data due to the nature of the discipline. Second, issues surrounding mentorship are discussed in detail.

Issues in Supervision

It is good practice to recognize the different characteristics of individual learners and to value all of the perspectives that all individuals bring with them to supervision. Many authors have reviewed scenarios thought to contribute to supportive learning communities. Programs such as the First Fellows, described by Brommer and Eisen (2006), have attempted to address diversity from the standpoint of participation in the sciences from undergraduate to professoriate levels. A similar work by Gooden, Leary, and Childress (1994) discussed an initiative aimed at increasing engagement of minority perspectives.

In a profession that faces a critical shortage of providers, it is imperative that quality training and supervision coexist. Clinical supervision in speech-language pathology is a cornerstone for successful development. Kirby, Morris, and Sullivan (2006) offered the challenge that "each generation of professionals should proceed the level of the last." They describe the styles of supervision as a clinician becomes more independent and transitions through the supervisory stages. It is important to adapt supervisory knowledge to the particular demands of the case as well as the student clinician, in an increasingly wider domain than ever before. Supervision of service delivery is a complex area of clinical practice. The opportunity to be a supervisor as well as a mentor comes with many distinct challenges.

Recently, the evolving dynamics of supervision and mentorship in other disciplines beyond speech-pathology (i.e., psychology and nursing) have been a topic of research and interest in the professional literature (Martino & Melcher, 2006; Owen & Solomon, 2006; Owen, Soloman, Mallozzi, Kline, & Wareham, 2007; Riordan & Kern, 1994; Rivera-Goba & Nieto, 2007; Sanchez & Reyes, 1999; Shilpi, 1998; Smith, 1989). In my opinion, supervision seems to have had greater attention in terms of objectified measurement. Presently, outcome measures of mentorship are becoming an area of active investigation due to an evolving need.

There are greater challenges due to the globalization of communication sciences and disorders and the clinical nature of the discipline, as well as technologic advances in delivery of services. Both specific job skills (supervision) and professional growth (mentorship) are challenges for the profession. This book attempts to bring these advances together into one volume to support and teach speech-language pathologists who currently or eventually want to serve a role in the development of professionals through clinical supervision.

In the pages to come, the supervisory process is explored both from the supervisor's and the student's position. Scenarios relating to the processes of supervision and the parameters to be included are brought together for the seasoned supervisor to reflect on and for the beginning supervisor to lean on in their new roles. The busy clinician may feel that research is not geared toward the needs of the practitioners. However, transformational research, such as applied in this book, is an information gathering approach geared to stimulate more productive relationships between research and practice.

Inherent in any practice that involves human dynamic variables as distinct as human communication, there are many challenges to distinguish. A wealth of information regarding the research methodology used to disentangle these factors exists and lies primarily in the realm of descriptive research. There is ample amount of agreement in conclusions by various researchers that supervision is a body of knowledge with principles and practices that should be learned alongside discipline-specific information. Using description of the literature, case study examples, and personal research, I hope to illuminate the area of research and supervision by accumulating some of the evidence bases for current and future practice.

Current Statistics

Prior to beginning a book on supervision, it is important to examine just who are the current players in the field of speech-language pathology and supervision. The following sections provide data on current ASHA demographics. As can be seen, these data also illustrate some of the relevant issues that are a running theme of the book, namely, the need for supervision and mentorship of nontraditional and multicultural students.

According to information compiled by ASHA as of 2007 (2008c), there were in excess of 127,000 members. The speech-language pathologists included in this number equal more than 106,000 holding their Certificate of Clinical Competence in speech-language pathology (commonly referred to as CCC-SLP). There also are members who choose not to hold certification, members in process of certification, as well as members holding dual certification in both speech-language pathology and audiology (although the latter number was only 1,256 at the end of the 2006 membership year). As the focus of this book is clinical supervision in speech-language pathology, the topic and training of professionals in audiology are not addressed.

Prior to the current licensure standards in our native state, many of us were trained and followed an identical course of study in "Speech and Hearing." The specialization that began in the early to mid-1970s has grown phenomenally to embrace subspecializations within speech and language as well as within adult and pediatric care.

Who Are the Current Speech-Language Pathologists?

Data compiled by ASHA report on demographics of newly joined members and nonmember certificate holders who were certified in 2004 and 2005. In 2004, out of a total number of 6,992 respondents, 1,621 individuals reporting ethnicity, 95.2% reported themselves as non-Hispanic or Latino, whereas only 4.8% reported Hispanic or Latino. In 2005, out of a total number of 7,510, 2,144 individuals reporting ethnicity shows a mild increase in proportion to 5.6% (Hispanic or Latino) and 94.4% (non-Hispanic). According to more recent statistics compiled in 2008, only approximately 7% of the ASHA membership are members of a racial minority, including non-member certificate holders and international affiliates (ASHA, 2008b). Of these, only a scant 3% of members identify themselves as being of Hispanic or Latino ethnicity (ASHA, 2008b). However, 12.5% of the United States population is identified as Hispanic and Latino in the census. This figure is in contrast to the 24.9% figure reported in the 2000 census as being of a racial minority background.

Although not completely applicable to our purposes, other statistics on age and gender demonstrate that the majority of providers that reported on age are within the age range of 35 to 44. Furthermore, only 4 to 5% of speech-language pathologists are male (ASHA, 2008b). For additional information about these figures, contact the ASHA's Surveys and Information unit. (A. M. Moxley, personal communication, July 29, 2010).

The supervision and mentorship of nontraditional individuals becomes increasingly important when you consider the needs of cases that may not necessarily match the demographic profiles of the clinicians that we are training. In response to this need, ASHA has put forth the Knowledge and Skills Needed by Speech-Language Pathologists and Audiologists to Provide Culturally and Linguistically Appropriate Services (ASHA, 2004c).

Initiatives to Encourage New Recruits

In a paper entitled, "Recruitment of Minorities into the Professions," Martino and Melcher (2006) of Xavier University of Louisiana reported that the majority of students do not recognize speech-language pathology as a potential career path, nor some of the intrinsic values that they are seeking to satisfy according to their general expressed career goals (i.e., desire to help others and job environments).

In response to these and many other relative issues, ASHA has established a number of initiatives, one of the most prominent being *Mentoring: The ASHA Gathering Place* (2004a). This is described as an online resource facilitating mentoring through guided experience. According to ASHA sources, 350 mentees and 550 mentors have since participated, with about one-half of the mentors being from a racial or ethnic minority background (K. Beverly-Ducker, personal communication, May 29, 2007). As can be gauged from the data presented, this presents a challenge to recruitment and retention of clinicians who are bilingually and biculturally proficient as well as to supervision and mentorship. As such, these vital issues are examined throughout this book.

Acknowledgments

I wish to thank Plural Publishing for asking me to write this book, in particular, Tom Murry and Stephanie Meissner. It has been a personal capstone on an already fulfilling career, which would not have been possible without the hard work and dedication of all the contributors and assistants who helped make this book a reality. I would like to thank the American-Speech-Language-Hearing Association for its willingness to dialogue with me and contribute organizational wisdom to the book. I wish to express my gratitude to the support and dedication of Fredericka Bell-Berti, Patrick Walden, Andrea Moxley, Tommie L. Robinson, Arlene Pietranon, Monica Gordon Pershey, Melanie Hudson, Susan Behrens, Blanca Vega, Tricia Molea-Santos, Mabel Lam, Ann Jablon, Teresa Signorelli, Melanie M. Domenech-Rodriguez, Valentina Concordia, Regina Volodarsky, Julia Nack, Celena S. Chong, and Alexa Lazzarotti. I also wish to thank all of the clients, teachers, clinical supervisors, and mentors who inspired me throughout my career. To my present colleagues, my work continues alongside you in our quest to deepen the understanding and appreciation of communication sciences and disorders. To Tanya Budilovskaya, I wish you the same satisfaction and fulfillment in your career as I have had in mine.

Contributors

Andrea "Deedee" Moxley, M.A., CCC-SLP
Associate Director
Multicultural Resources
ASHA Student to Empowered Professional (S.T.E.P.) Mentoring
  Coach
American Speech-Language-Hearing Association
Rockville, Maryland
Chapter 9

Patrick R. Walden, PhD, CCC-SLP
Assistant Professor of Communication Sciences and Disorders
St. John's University
New York, New York
Chapter 10

ASHA Interviews

Interviews with distinguished professionals in the field of speech-language pathology were obtained for the purposes of this book. Interviews were conducted with Tommie L. Robinson, the current president of the American Speech-Language-Hearing Association, as well as Dr. Arlene Pietranton, Executive Director of the American Speech-Language-Hearing Association. Both individuals reflected on personal and professional experiences with regard to mentorship, personal views and beliefs regarding mentorship, and how it should be conducted. The interviews below were conducted in different modalities based on the interviewee's preference, thus reflecting the different styles in which they are presented. The author wishes to thank both Dr. Robinson and Dr. Pietranton for their time and generosity in contribution to this book, as well as for sharing their extensive experience and expertise.

Tommie L. Robinson Jr., PhD, CCC-SLP, 2009–2010 ASHA President

1. *Did you have a mentor?*
I had thousands of them. Well, maybe not thousands, but I have had a lot of mentors over both my time as a student and in my professional life. I have relied on different mentors for different things. For research, for administration, teaching, and for personal advice.

2. *How did you pick your mentor?*
I really didn't do it as a plan. It just happened naturally. I had admiration for the person or they showed an interest in me, or I saw them in a less formal setting and got to know them. Then it evolved into a mentoring relationship.

3. *Did someone select you to mentor? How did they help you?*
During my days in graduate school in Mississippi when I was study-ing for my Master's degree, one of my professors, Dr. Thomas Crowe, asked me to come to his office and meet with him. He had just returned from an ASHA meeting in Washington, DC, and had spent time with a number of African American leaders in our professions and was very impressed by them. He decided that I had the potential to be a leader, like them, and told me so. He said, "Tommie, I want you to go to Howard and get your PhD." He was a person that I admired and respected so I decided to follow his advice. Later on, I presented a lecture to a class as a part of my graduate assistantship and he overheard some students talking about how much they had enjoyed my topic. He said to me, "One day you will be ASHA president." He took me under his wing. I was like a third son to him. I could ask him for advice on a whole range of issues.

4. *Have you mentored students and/or professionals?*
I have a number of students who regularly call me for advice and I would like to think that I am also a mentor to colleagues in my work setting. I do have friends who call me on a regular basis to talk and to get advice.

5. *How do you mentor?*
It usually grows out of a relationship, like working on a thesis, and then the student asks for advice and the relationship grows and develops. Since I have had a number of mentors, I am conscious of the mentoring process and work to develop mentoring relationships with my students. The process is both natural and planned. For exam-ple, I might be asked to give a talk somewhere and I can't do it because of my schedule so I'll suggest a colleague where I think such an opportunity would be good for them to move their career forward. I won't just suggest the person, I'll explain to the requestor why I think this is a good fit for their needs. I will also introduce students or professional colleagues to others who I think can help them grow.

6. *What made your experiences successful?*
The key is honesty and trust. You must have a good relationship with your mentee. Good mentoring relationships start from that foundation.

7. *What made your experiences unsuccessful?*

I had one experience with a person who was trying to mentor me, but I felt they had an ulterior motive. I felt this person was giving me advice that would help them, and was not genuine. The mentoring relationship never got off the ground.

8. *Do you think there is confusion among the terms of mentoring/supervisor/role model?*

Yes, I think there can be some confusion and they are not the same thing. A supervisor can be a mentor, but a role model can be someone you never met, but just admire. Supervisors and mentors have to be active participants. Certainly, some of these roles do overlap.

9. *Do cultural/gender differences affect the success of the process?*

Short answer, no. I guess maybe they can, but in my experience, it's not that important to the role, that is, it is not that important to be of the same culture or gender in order to have a good mentor/mentee relationship. The most important thing is the synergy between the two individuals. I guess it can help, but I certainly don't think it is a must.

10. *How do you define mentoring?*

Mentoring is when someone takes an interest in you for the sole purpose of making you better at what you do. They give you guidance and advice designed to make you a better professional, a better person.

Arlene A. Pietranton, PhD, CAE, ASHA Executive Director

1. *Did you have a mentor?*

Dr. Pietranton indicated that she has had several caring individuals in the course of her professional life who were invaluable in their generous spirit and example. She mentioned that there was never an explicit articulation of mentorship, but a mutual atmosphere of candid communication at different phases in her work.

She stated that there is not a one-size-fits-all answer to mentorship. There are many factors with dynamic interplay including factors such as learning styles and culture. She stated that mentorship and supervision are not the same but have common characteristics.

Importantly, Dr. Pietranton stated that the ASHA National Office employs a model of "coaching" (vs. "supervision") in which there is mutual responsibility to enhance the goals of organization. This language and concept assists in clarifying the focus on the fact that the "coachee's" success is also a part of the coach's success. A collaborative model that is centered on the concept that the coach's "job" is to help the individuals who report to him.

2. *Can you describe situations in which you have served as a mentor and what are your practices as a mentor?*

In all of her formal and informal mentoring experiences, Dr. Pietranton emphasizes that the goal of the mentor should be to ask oneself, "What can I do to help this person?" An additional and important factor, Dr. Pietranton cautions that mentorship must be individualized. In some scenarios, setting goals and pathways may be extremely important and appropriate, whereas in others, mentorship may take on a different focus. Some individuals may benefit from advice to, "do something you care about with passion and energy, and that passion and energy will be noticed." In all cases, the focus of the mentor is on the benefit and goals of the mentee.

Dr. Pietranton stresses the words of "candor" and "authenticity" in her description of the type of optimal communication between mentors and mentees.

She affirms that the activities of a mentor in this regard may include and are not limited to: listening, advising, providing opportunities, including mentee in one's work, introducing mentee to other, and many other activities.

In describing an experience in which practices of supervision and mentorship were not optimal, Dr. Pietranton mentions respect for the mentee especially in the actual clinic arena where clients or third parties are present. In fact, she shared a preference to not interrupt a session unless actual "harm" is being done. She notes that many times, a situation may be handled more effectively and that the supervisor-mentor can inform the novice professional away from the actual client contact session.

Dr. Pietranton and the author concurred that the type of supervisory education that committed supervisors are seeking in today's learning place actually helps improve the communication styles of supervisors to handle situations. This was not part of the traditional clinical and theoretical education of speech-language pathologists, hence potentially decreasing the type of scenario presented above.

ASHA has many initiatives related to mentorship in addition to the S.T.E.P. program is the MARC program, the SPARC program, and the Office of Multicultural Affairs. The profession is benefiting from these initiatives as exhibited on many levels of membership and leadership in ASHA.

3. *Any other factors that affect the success of the process?*
Dr. Pietranton mentions that suitability for an effective mentoring team may come from many sources. In fact, she states that individuals who look at things differently may have a lot to share and learn from each other. There are many factors, formal and informal, that may support a strong mentoring match. Personality and cultural backgrounds do not have to be the same but can be complementary and serve to facilitate new perspectives.

She mentions that a strong mentoring component to a work setting is a very forward-thinking and proactive choice to make. It can decrease from a "wait and see" attitude. Therefore, there are potential benefits beyond strength and growth of the mentor and mentee that extend to success of a given environment in prevention of difficult situations.

Dr. Pietranton defines a good mentor as an "individual who is willing to be in the relationship strictly for the good of the mentee," although in the process, the mentor may learn a good deal as well!

This book is lovingly dedicated to my children,
Christopher and Elizabeth,
and the memory of my husband, Raymond James Carozza,
who accompanied me on my journey
through life and in my work.
He was with me the day that my PhD was conferred,
and knew that I was going to write a book about my career
in speech-language pathology. He would be so proud.

SECTION I

Understanding the Issues

CHAPTER 1

Introduction: Definitions and Introduction to Concepts

Supervisors serve as the keepers of the faith and the mentors of the young. Theirs is a quiet profession that combines the discipline of science with the aesthetic creativity of art ... It is a curious paradox that at their best they are the least visible.

Ann Alonso, 'The Quiet Profession'

Introduction to Concepts

As stated in ASHA's position statement on clinical supervision in speech-language pathology (ASHA, 2008a), "clinical supervision (also called clinical teaching or clinical education) is a distinct area of practice in speech-language pathology and is an essential component in the education of students and the continual professional growth of speech-language pathologists" (p. 1). Clinical supervision also is a collaborative process, with shared responsibility for many of the activities throughout the supervisory experience. The companion document, *Knowledge and Skills Needed by Speech-Language Pathologists Providing Clinical Supervision* (ASHA, 2008b) delineates areas of competence, and the position statement, *Clinical Supervision in Speech-Language Pathology* (ASHA, 2008a) affirms the role of supervision within the profession.

Clinical supervision is an integral component of the profession of speech-language pathology and has important implications for the education of future clinicians, the continuous professional growth of speech-language pathologists, and, most importantly, the clients. As stated above, basic supervision is a collaborative process between the student and the supervisor, which is meant to facilitate an exchange of knowledge and ideas as well as to help budding clinicians develop their own clinical styles and cultivate their own ideas and reflections on their clients.

Just as Anderson (1988) discusses the continuum of supervision, there also is a continuum of supervision and mentorship. For purposes of organization, supervision is discussed in the first section of the book and mentorship in the latter part. Although the lines often are blurred between the two, a supervisor generally is considered the senior of two individuals and concerned with task demands and performance during work hours in a designated setting. A mentor, on the other hand, may seek to develop the employee's competence not only in one particular setting, but also to prepare them for work challenges in different environments and to seek highest possible personal and professional competencies. An in-depth discussion about mentorship follows in the later portions of the book.

Rewards and Challenges of Supervision

The practice of supervising another individual engaged in service delivery calls on a number of different skill sets and professional competencies. The professional competencies explored throughout this book include an understanding of interpersonal communication styles, cultural and linguistic factors, personal resilience, and sensitivity to social power. These are illustrated through the use of clinical case scenarios and data from real-life supervisory dialogues.

As with any professional discipline, supervision presents its own unique set of issues and challenges. A range of personal and professional issues and challenges which may hinder one's ability to perform their duties as a supervisor are discussed in detail. On the other hand, supervision can be a very rewarding and satisfying experience for both the supervisor and the supervisee, especially when approached with the right mindset and armed with the proper knowledge and skills. There are distinct motivations associated with supervision, as described in an ASHA (n.d.) publication and detailed below:

Top 10 Reasons to Supervise a Student

1. Develop and recruit future employees.
2. Stay current—learn what students are learning.
3. Share your expertise with future SLP's.
4. Establish a relationship with university programs.
5. Teach future SLP's to advocate for SLP services.
6. Introduce students to interdisciplinary team building.
7. Feel good about giving back to the profession.
8. Develop your mentoring and supervisory skills.
9. Enhance your clinical skills by teaching someone else.
10. Leave a legacy.

ASHA Resources

The field of speech-language pathology has done a tremendous amount to support the knowledge of supervision despite the fact that it is not a distinct area of practice recognized by ASHA as of yet. Nevertheless, ASHA has provided clinicians with numerous essential resources. The guidelines for clinical supervision are stated in the membership and certification handbook provided by ASHA (http://www.asha.org/about/membership-certification/). Supervisors also have a companion guideline in the Clinical Fellowship Supervisors

Responsibilities, which is available via ASHA (http://www.asha.org/certification/CFSupervisors.htm). Additionally, the Special Interest Division 11 of the American Speech-Language Hearing Association (http://www.asha.org/members/divs/div_11.htm) is the centerpiece of information dissemination pertaining to supervision and related topics. The work of individual leaders in supervision, such as Newman (2001, 2008) and Victor (2001) have made significant contributions to advance the study in this field.

It is of interest to note that, although we have membership figures, it is difficult to determine the number of active supervisors at any given time. This partially may be accounted for by the relative fluidity of supervisory assignments in many settings. For example, an individual may not be a full-time supervisor and therefore may identify primarily as a speech-language pathologist, obscuring their supervisory roles. Nevertheless, part-time or full-time supervision requires a sound basis in clinical teaching.

Overview of History in Supervision Research

Speech-language pathology itself is a relatively young profession. The American Speech-Language-Hearing Association was established only in 1925 and has since grown exponentially. Its mission is to support and empower speech-language pathologists. As the profession is relatively new, both the practice and principles of therapy and supervision are also still developing. However, with recent technologic and scientific advancements, these changes are taking place at an increasingly rapid rate. As a result, the roles and responsibilities of speech-language pathologists will continue to expand.

Those clinicians that enter supervision are called on to learn not only the discipline-specific knowledge but also additional competencies in clinical education (i.e., supervision). In order to be an effective supervisor, it is important to know the foundation of this area. All supervisors should be knowledgable about the history of supervisory education as well as current research trends, starting with models of supervision as per Jean Anderson (1988) through the trend toward evidence-based practice in supervision (Dollaghan, 2007). I believe there is a need to stimulate this awareness on the part of new professionals through attention in our educational programs, individual training, and continuing education. This will become more urgent with the advancements in the field as well as the globalization of speech-language pathology consumers and providers.

It is interesting to note that, close to 30 years ago, supervision was considered a neglected component of the profession, as addressed in Turton's (1973) book, which cites models of peer supervision, reflective practice, and the case study approach to supervision, some of which are discussed in greater detail throughout this book. Highlights of the history are discussed below, including several current methods of supervisory evaluative strategies, such as traditional, group, peer, verbal, written, self-reflective (i.e., conversational analysis and metapragmatic awareness), as well as immediate and delayed feedback.

Foundational Models of Supervision

The study of supervision has a strong history, much of it building on Jean Anderson's seminal work (1988) and Dowling's work (1979, 1983, 1987), among others. Anderson (1988) proposed a continuum model for supervision, which recognizes that there are stages of growth that require modification of the input from the supervisor and the supervisee at different stages. Anderson's (1988) three stages of the continuum include the Evaluation-Feedback, Transition, and Self-Supervision Stages. According to this model, supervisees move back and forth along the continuum throughout their professional training and careers, assuming more or less responsibility for their clinical and supervisory skills. Anderson (1988) was one of the first to discuss differences in communication styles, and how these may impact the interactions of the student-supervisor dyad. The original model can be further expanded to include learner differences, such as those explored in this book.

Dowling (1979, 1983, 1987) proposed an alternative to the traditional one-on-one supervision methodology by introducing the concept of teaching clinic conferences, a group supervisory approach. This approach was based on models of supervision used frequently in counseling and teacher education. It is a very structured form of peer group supervision in which one participant, the demonstration clinician, presents a videotape of treatment to the group for observation, analysis, evaluation, and discussion. It was used to examine the perceptions of supervisor and peer behavior. This concept was later expanded on by A. Lynn Williams (1995), who incorporated concepts of collegiality and self-supervision into the original model. These concepts build on the notion that clinicians can learn not only from "top-down" models of supervision, but also from each other and a team approach.

Mawdsley and Scudder (1989) brought forth a different perspective. They developed the Integrative Task-Maturity Model of Supervision (ITMMS), an eight-step supervisory structure. This model was developed to help supervisors determine a supervisee's task-maturity level, adopt the appropriate supervisory style, and decide which supervisory techniques to use. It drew on an initial assessment of the supervisee's maturity as defined by their ability to act independently. Students were rated according to the following criteria: Input from supervisor yielded no measurable change in behavior, specific input was needed to yield exact change, general instruction only was needed, and, at the final stage, student functioned independently with no input required. Depending on maturity level, supervisory style was established and planned with the supervisee, followed by a strategy of observation and instruction, teaching and learning sequence, and a planned conference and analysis with renewed planning for the next cycle. This model was unique in that it took into account the important concept of personal maturity, which was not accounted for previously. This represents the accountability for individual differences, of which supervisors should be cognizant.

Current Trends in Models of Supervision

The consideration of individual differences is important to supervision models. One creative way in which to take these differences into account is the methodology of supervision described by McCready and Raleigh (2009). In the work of reflective practice as applied to supervision and speech-pathology (which is explored in later chapters), the use of narratives has become an all important tool to provide structure for personal and professional growth. The authors contend that teaching involves a deep understanding of self. Clinical supervisors may create a philosophy of supervision that starts through the instrument of self-reflective narratives in which personal belief systems and values are explored.

This practice may lead to a deeper understanding of sense of self and an appreciation for individual differences. Insight from this article further can be extended to student clinicians and supervisors by writing personal narratives and/or a written documentation (i.e., journal) of their unfolding development through their training. Additionally, there is room to consider a philosophy about teaching supervision, which is a potential outgrowth for experienced clinicians. This is among one of the current trends in promoting effective supervision.

Another reflective approach, discussed later in the text (Behrens et al., 2007), centers around the examination of supervisory exchanges from the standpoint of conversational analysis. They contended that there is a need for heightened awareness of conversational patterns in learning environments. This relates back to the notion earlier addressed by Anderson (1988) of differences in communicative styles and how they may play a role in the supervisory interaction. As an extension, the work of Behrens and Jablon (2008) can be used as a tool in supervisory education to heighten awareness of what is being communicated and how it is being transmitted. Excerpts from this research are provided later in the text as examples for teaching. The science of how to supervise and how to receive supervision is advanced through this research outcome, due to a shared appreciation of effective communication.

In this group of studies, conducted by Behrens et al. (2007), student-supervisor conversational dyads were analyzed using conversational analysis and metapragmatic awareness techniques. Assessment included judgment of overall communicative success, judgment of aspects such as the ability to express oneself, the ability to be understood, and negotiation skills. In addition to metapragmatic analysis which concerns the speaker's own perception of his or her own conversational style, this author's colleagues explore, in other work, speaker perceptions of communicative effectiveness in other work (Behrens & Jablon, 2008).

Current work on a related topic, pertaining to written as opposed to oral narratives, was conducted by Meilijson and Katzenberger (2009). The two authors analyzed the content of written reflections prepared by first and second year students in speech-language pathology. They conducted a qualitative analysis of the narratives in terms of whether there was an attempt to return to the original experience written about, attention to feelings, and evaluation of the experience. The results indicated that text length increased with level of learning. As students matured, they tended to use deeper reflective strategies.

There is evidence to suggest that the use of narratives may be used to evaluate students during the clinical education process. I have adapted this strategy in having my interns describe how clients evolved over time and how they perceived themselves to change throughout the course of therapeutic sessions. This notion of reflective practice as an integral aspect of evidence-based practice in supervision is discussed in detail in Chapter 7.

A recent study conducted by Ho and Whitehill (2009) compared individual supervision strategies. The researchers compared verbal immediate feedback with delayed written feedback. Results showed that students perceived advantages and disadvantages with both methods. Overall, students in the immediate verbal feedback group received significantly higher ratings in clinic evaluation than those in the delayed written feedback group. The immediate verbal feedback group also scored higher on self-evaluation. The authors concluded that studies of clinical education should be intensified to identify strategies that improve supervisor-supervisee communication.

All of the studies above highlight the fact that discipline-specific knowledge in and of itself is insufficient to guarantee quality supervision. The supervisor should have background knowledge of theoretical constructs and clinical approaches to supervision that have proven successful. This then allows the supervisor to enter the supervisory role armed with the knowledge and skills that have been acquired through scientific study of supervision. This establishes the initial basis for his or her own evidence-based approach to supervision.

The tools of self-awareness, respect for individual differences, and reflection shed new light on professional supervision. As evident in the studies above, many inter- and intrapersonal variables play a role in the dynamics of supervision. As such, supervisors should be cognizant of these factors, and use the strategies available from the literature as well as make modifications as their practice dictates. This can contribute to both personal and professional growth of the student and the supervisor throughout their careers. Currently, a great deal of literature focuses on the increasing responsibilities of supervisors, updated models, and the need to support an increase of clinical educators (McAllister, 2005; McAllister, Higgs, & Smith, 2008; Newman, 2001).

This chapter highlighted some of the important concepts, definitions, and background information necessary to begin thinking about and understanding our role as clinical supervisors. We examined some of the potential benefits and rewards that come with being a supervisor and provided the reader with some excellent resources for further reading. We also highlighted some of the salient history of clinical supervision, from early foundation models proposed by pioneers in the field to more current trends. All of the work conducted in this field to date has paved the way for the future and new directions.

What's Next?

In the following chapter, we examine some of the current issues prevailing in supervision research. We also consider some novel approaches to addressing these issues using current research. Some of the variables influencing the supervisor-supervisee relationship are discussed and illustrated using case study examples.

Reflective Assignment

Create a list of relevant words that come to mind when thinking about the supervision process. These may include feelings, concepts, personal attributes, qualities you hope to cultivate in supervisees and/or in yourself, perception of roles and responsibilities, and so forth. Think about how each of these would play out during the supervisory process. In the first column, write your own words. In the second column, write words that you think a supervisee may generate. I have started you off with a few examples:

Supervisor's Words	Supervisee's Words
Experience	Anxiety
Growth	Challenge
Guidance	Feedback
Support	Professionalism

CHAPTER 2

Issues in Supervision Research: A Case Study Approach

Tell me and I forget, teach me and I remember,
involve me and I learn.

Benjamin Franklin

Supervision Models

This chapter is an extension on the literature of the models of supervision described in the previous chapter, which were developed through empirical as well as case study research. These include the models developed by Anderson (1977), Dowling (1979), Mawdsley and Scudder (2005), McCrea and Brasseur (2003), McCready and Raleigh (2009), Moses and Shapiro (1996), and Williams (1995). This chapter attempts to integrate the following: empirical research in supervision models, case study research, and challenges in supervision, particularly those that arise from cultural differences.

These models serve to provide us with a broad basis for understanding and applying the principles of supervision and have important implications for the field. However, these models frequently are very broad in scope and may not always account for all of the day-to-day nuances that arise in supervision. Other limitations exist in all research protocols when the results cannot be readily applied outside of the population studied. There are many factors for this, such as methodologic constraints, including subject matching, procedure selection, and other variables. This precludes a comparative review or true meta-analysis according to definition. However, these issues are unavoidable in this line of research.

The issues presented in this chapter include cross-cultural differences, needs of nontraditional students, communication breakdowns, and other current concerns facing practitioners. Each of these issues is presented with the use of case studies. Thus, before we begin to explore each of these issues, the following provides an overview of the case study approach.

The Case Study Approach: Operational Shifts and Changes of Assumptions

Supervision has been studied through various approaches, with case study exemplars being a highly informative format. This format allows the teacher-trainer to take multiple perspectives. Individual case studies can be used to instruct clinical teaching and supervision in special needs cases, which is central to this chapter. The case study approach examines clinical interactions using an in-depth approach on an individual basis. Case study approaches are one way to bridge the gap between the breadth of knowledge and the depth of experience in order to attempt to anticipate clinical conflicts before they arise.

Although case study single-subject design has inherent limitations on generalizability, a study of atypical cases may be a good starting point by which to systematize observations. Case studies are used extensively in education, business, and legal research and have been used in speech-language pathology. In the field of supervision, case-teaching scenarios are an established teaching tool. It is designed to prepare the student and clinical trainer for exposure to situations that they may not have previously anticipated in the educational setting. Thus, studies of supervisory scenarios that involve complicated or extenuating factors are important to study as this is at the forefront of society given more diverse providers and caseloads. Case studies allow us to examine a model against the actual practice. According to French (1997), a case study approach has been useful in studying the author's interaction with a speech-pathology assistant. Although both the generalizations of the findings and the number of studies using the case study approach are limited, research in supervision at all levels may be greatly enhanced by increased use of this methodology.

In light of this, exemplary case study descriptions are used to highlight specific challenges that may be encountered in supervision. Formal case study/single subject design ideally is approached with a specific supervisory research question in mind (i.e., effect of immediate versus delayed feedback on an individual student's perceived confidence). Nevertheless, informal teaching vignettes (as seen below) are a standard teaching tool and extensions may be possible by employing specific research questions. An effective supervisor may be interested in using standard research design to uncover possible factors in how his or her practices impact workplace issues. By combining factual and experiential data, the perspective of the reader is broadened, and the continuum of supervision is extended to include novel problem-based learning. Initially, targeted observations in the form of the assignment that follows this chapter would be a useful place by which to begin, in addition to other protocols found in this book.

The following scenarios highlight areas of concern to supervisors; namely, cultural differences, application of textbook knowledge, communication breakdown, issues of clinical competence, and the needs of nontraditional students. This is followed by a narrative of a nontraditional student as she describes her perspective.

Case Studies

Global Perspectives

Tricia Molea-Santos, MS, CCC-SLP

A. Cultural Differences

"You have to think harder!" Ms. Smith, the clinical supervisor, said to one of her students. She pointed her finger at Janet's forehead. Janet took a quick glance around her. The nurses at the

station were trying to hide their shock by looking down at their patient files. Silence was deafening.

Janet said to herself, "How could I let my supervisor know that what she's saying was never taught in class that way?" Janet was the only Asian student in her class. Being Asian, she was always brought up not to speak back toward superiors. Little did Ms. Smith know, Janet was among the few straight A students in her class.

Culture is an important aspect in clinical supervision and is one of the primary issues that faces the new supervisor and student, as exemplified in the vignette above. Most Asian cultures, for example, show respect for elders or superiors by avoiding direct confrontation. Other cultures, on the other hand, stress the importance of "speaking one's mind." It is suggested that a presupervision session be held to determine the best means of communication between the student and supervisor. This is the central point of the later chapter discussion.

B. Real-World Application of Textbook Knowledge

"That is not the information they gave us in class!" Hillary defiantly stood up and reached for her textbook. She flipped through the pages very briskly, stopped at a specific page, and pointed out the paragraph. Her supervisor, Ms. Smith, was surprised by her student's reaction. Ms. Smith was warned by other clinical supervisors about this straight A student who "always fought for her grade" in the past. How could she tell Hillary that clinical practice was beyond merely reading books?

All supervisors have heard students ask how they will use textbook knowledge in the real world and how their work as clinicians reflects personal knowledge. Some supervision scenarios require the student clinician to think beyond the four walls of the classroom. Students should know that not everything taught in class necessarily applies to the different clinical scenarios. Thus, it is the clinical supervisor's task to challenge the student to find the balance between books and the clinical world. There are many cases in which student clinicians require real "life skills" before they can approach the challenge of a handicapped child in a family or how the issue of a stroke disabling the family breadwinner will devastate family relationships. Some things cannot be taught and supervisors cannot be all things to all people. However, bringing real-life scenarios and case studies to class discussions can be enlightening and helpful.

C. Communication Breakdown

Robert turned to his client's family as soon as the test was finished. He decided this was his case and that he need not consult his supervisor, Ms. McGraw. "Ms. Valdes, your husband passed the test! He is not aspirating on any of the barium we gave him. He should be free to eat anything at home, given necessary feeding precautions."

Ms. McGraw was surprised by Robert's misinterpretation of the videofluoroscopy study. She was more stunned by his quickness to respond without consulting her. How would Ms. McGraw inform her clients of Robert's mistake without putting him to shame?

There are cases in which the student will misread or incorrectly interpret test results. These may have important implications for the client and family as in the case above involving feeding issues and medical clearance. Student clinicians as well as supervisors should be in close communication in all situations, especially those with immediate medical implications. In all cases, communication is always the best solution to breakdowns in student and clinical supervisor relationships. Once an avenue for expressing feedback and opinions has been established, miscommunication rarely occurs. Good interpersonal skills and establishment of routine behaviors are skills that a disciplined supervisor must model and adhere to in his or her role as a supervisor.

D. Issues of Clinical Competence

*"Could I be the one to add the speech valve on my next patient?"
Sarah turned to her supervisor. "Sure, go ahead. I just need to
make a phone call. I'll be right back," replied Mr. Martel.*

    *It wasn't 2 minutes when Mr. Martel frantically ran from the
nurses' station. The ICU nurses called a Code Red. The patient
turned blue and had trouble breathing. Sarah was asked to leave
the room. The attending physician was furious. Across the hall,
Mr. Martel heard the doctor yell at Sarah, "If I were you, I would
not show my face in the ICU anymore. You nearly killed my
patient!" Sarah failed her externship and was asked to repeat
another semester at the hospital.*

Clinical supervisors are liable for the mistakes of their students.
This may be self-explanatory, yet in some clinical settings, students
still take the full blame and responsibility for these clinical mistakes. It is the role of the supervisor to stay with a student to the
point that a student is fully independent in any assigned function.
The role of side-by-side clinical cooperation in the care of all
patients cannot be undermined and should be carefully monitored
and maintained.

Nontraditional Student: "Emily and Dr. Haskins: Classroom Expectations, Pragmatics, and Clinical Acumen"

Susan Behrens, Ph.D.
Professor of Communication Sciences and Disorders, Marymount
Manhattan College

Linda Carozza, Ph.D., CCC-SLP
Assistant Professor of Communication Sciences and Disorders, St.
John's University

Case study research conducted by the present author and her colleague, Susan Behrens, (2007) consisted of an original research

project that included a scenario of an atypical supervision situation involving challenges in the supervisee's clinical dispositions. This case study reflects one of the challenges not heretofore described in the literature, namely, an individual whose clinical abilities were compromised by a previously undiagnosed disorder, and who ultimately was not fit to study as a clinical practitioner. In addition to cross-cultural factors, it is my experience that one of the most important issues in supervision is dealing with the needs of nontraditional students. This is further discussed at the chapter conclusion. The following is an excerpt from, "Emily and Dr. Haskins: Classroom Expectations, Pragmatics, and Clinical Acumen" (Behrens & Carozza, 2007).[1] See http://www.sciencecases.org/emily/emily.asp for the complete case study.

> The case study profiles a hard-working student of clinical psychology with good grades who, nonetheless, does not possess the clinical skills necessary to work in the field. In addition, the student's placement on the autistic spectrum is never fully revealed by the student. Thus, professors are ill informed and not prepared to deal with the student. They may eventually become more informed through such methods as discourse and conversational analysis; discussions with senior supervisors; and assignment of more than one supervisor to a student. In other words, supervision should be elevated as a science. In addition, educators could be better trained to identify and work with students on the autistic spectrum ... Perhaps an alternative track could be presented to students who do not pass a mid-program assessment or clinical fitness test. Students in the allied health fields need to be aware of the full array of skills necessary for successful entrance into their chosen field. (Behrens & Carozza, 2007)

Acknowledgments. This case was developed with support from the National Science Foundation under CCLI Award #0341279. Any opinions, findings and conclusions or recommendations expressed

---

[1]Portions of this article were originally published by the National Center for Case Study Teaching in Science (NCCSTS) under the title, "Emily and Dr. Haskins: Classroom Expectations, Pragmatics, and Clinical Acumen" by Susan Behrens and Linda Carozza. Copyright held by the NCCSTS. Used with permission.

in this material are those of the author(s) and do not necessarily reflect the views of the National Science Foundation. Date Posted: 02/06/07 nas

A Self-Study

Mabel Lam
Graduate student, Nova Southeastern University

The following self-study has been contributed by Mabel Lam, a foreign-born speech-language pathology student.

I feel it is important to remove subjectivity from supervisory feedback. Newman (2008) indicated the following points to establish and maintain an effective working relationship:

1. Clinical educators need to recognize the power differential and be sensitive to it. The supervisory relationship is a unique one, and because of the fragility of the relationship, it usually is not beneficial to exert power when working with the supervisee.

2. An atmosphere where learning is supported should be provided.

3. The supervisee should feel comfortable in presenting thoughts and ideas relative to clinical challenges.

4. On the other side of the supervisory relationship, it may not be healthy to develop a close "friendship" with the supervisee.

5. The supervisee needs to understand that the supervisor is a teacher and too much social comfort may not provide for a situation where the supervisor can evaluate performance independently of the relationship.

6. A balance where the supervisor and supervisee are "friendly" and where the relationship is one of mutual respect and support is optimal.

7. Open and ongoing communication between the supervisor and the supervisee is central to the success of the supervisory relationship.

Based on points 1, 2, 3, and 7, it is suggested that the supervisor should not exert power when working with the supervisee, a supportive learning atmosphere is recommended, and the supervisor should allow the supervisee to present thoughts and ideas. An open and ongoing communication pattern between the supervisor and the supervisee contributes to a successful working relationship. Therefore, the supervisor's subjectivity may work against the above requirements. For example, if the supervisor criticizes the supervisee's words and behavior based on her subjective point of view without considering the supervisee's point of view and personal preference (including personality and cultural background), a supportive learning atmosphere will be disrupted and an open communication pattern will be thwarted.

On the other hand, according to points 4, 5, and 6, it is suggested that a professional boundary should be established between the supervisor and the supervisee. A close, friendly relationship is unhealthy because too much social comfort will affect a fair and objective evaluation. The roles of teacher and student should be clearly defined, although in some cases the supervisor and the supervisee are friends or coworkers. For example, if the supervisor overlooks the supervisee's errors because of their friendly relationship, it is also due to the supervisor's subjectivity because he or she cannot stay objective in evaluating the person's performance and the situation.

Cross-Cultural Differences

What makes someone "difficult" to supervise? It may reside in cross-cultural differences. Because we reside in a vastly diverse multicultural society, we are bound to work with individuals from different cultural and/or linguistic backgrounds at some point. Students and supervisors who come from different cultural and/or linguistic backgrounds may have very different ideas as to what constitutes acceptable interpersonal behaviors, communicative styles, forms of address, and so forth. Assigning readings written by authors outside of the field of speech-language pathology may serve as helpful guides on how to respectfully communicate and navigate in a diverse world (see a reader-friendly review from Aguilar [2006] *Ouch! That Stereotype Hurts*, printed by Walk the Talk Co.).

Another solution that has been proposed based on a series of research is the peer-supervision model. This particular approach is received favorably by new clinicians and actually exceeded their expectations when trialed in a New York City undergraduate speech-language pathology training program. The seminal work of Dr. Lynn Williams (1995), an ASHA Fellow as well as a professor at East Tennessee University, indicates that this model is very helpful, particularly with students of minority backgrounds. After working with it, Dr. Williams has expressed support for this model of supervision as a strategy to the current author in her work with multicultural student clinicians.

Multicultural issues in supervision also have been discussed and analyzed extensively throughout the literature. In 1989, Shapiro and Moses proposed a practical and self-described "collegial" model of practices to apply in the diverse environments of the public school system. A decade later, Moses and Shapiro (1996) reported on a methodology for education of student clinicians at different levels of development. This was a major contribution to the study of "how to supervise" in that the expectations differ as students gain perspective and skill sets improve. Problem-solving domains, including assuming perspectives, considering the range of variables and generating multiple solutions are all developmental processes in clinical learning. These issues are compounded when multicultural factors are added to the clinical training environment.

It is of extreme importance to note that intercultural mentorship is gaining the attention of academics in all disciplines. Crutcher (2007) notes in her guide to best practices that the dyads do not necessarily have to come from the same or similar backgrounds, but do need to carefully explore the implications of their differences. This is juxtaposed with the need to establish and maintain good boundaries. Inappropriate distancing on the part of the mentor will cause the mentee to withdraw. It is imperative that all teachers be trained on how to mentor so we can support all our students, regardless of the area of instruction. It not only diversifies but democratizes education. As most of the mentors do not come from the ranks of a racial or ethnic minority, there must be groundwork to make cross-cultural mentoring work.

Roman and Carozza (2007) brought the issue of the need to increase representation of the minorities in the speech-language pathology profession to the professional community at large. The authors described the problems in the pipeline leading to graduate education. There is a dearth of Spanish-speaking professionals to meet the needs of academically challenged children. In general, Hispanics also are behind other ethnic groups in achieving higher education. Minority professionals are called on to increase public awareness and help other minorities achieve and succeed academically.

Blake-Beard, Murrell, and Thomas (2006) wrote a paper called, "Unfinished Business: The Impact of Race on Understanding Mentoring Relationships," which discussed this aspect of the mentoring process. From the standpoint of a clinician who has been on both sides of this situation, the material that Blake-Beard, Murrell, and Thomas (2006) produced is on target. There appears to be a need to actually train mentorship in education, similar to how we train the clinical portion of speech-language pathology. Supervisory competencies should be demonstrated satisfactorily to achieve fairness to both supervisor and supervisee. Only then can the dyad enter into a solid foundation of shared clinical work.

One of the most relevant works that has implications to the cultural aspects described in this book is an article written by Staub (2009) entitled "Facilitating Cultural Fluency for a Multicultural Society." Being that multiculturalism is an important facet of our society, it plays a great role in workplace practice as well. Staub (2009) argues that supervisors in all areas of clinical work have a practical and ethical responsibility to train workers to be culturally fluent, which he describes as a process to attain self-awareness as a means of establishing "responsive, reciprocal, and respectful" relationships. It is necessary for all parties to evaluate themselves in their progress toward becoming culturally competent. Included later in this chapter are real-life case scenarios of student clinicians' experience with supervision and some thought-provoking discussions concerning the relevant issues and areas detailed above.

The concept of career mentorship extends from the time a young student is in high school perhaps contemplating a possible career path for the first time through to the time when a person is settled in the middle stages of a career. Academic life requires emotional and educational vigor. The need for stamina to develop and maintain a career in a challenging field such as human communication is certain. The support of internal mentors (maybe family members) to external mentors (past and present colleagues, perhaps paid counselors, or coaches) is integral to career satisfaction and maintenance of the intellectual curiosity that drives these career paths.

The field of speech and language pathology depends on the growth and nurturance of newly minted PhDs to take the place of retiring faculty in the university settings that serve as the training ground for the master's level degree required to practice in the discipline. Recruiting and retaining talent is a mainstay of university success in all fields. In speech-language pathology, there is a need for increased representation of diverse faculty to meet population and demographic changes.

Carozza (2002) described the issues relative to minorities, particularly Hispanics in higher education. At stake is a future generation of scholars committed to studying communication issues in general, as well as those that are generated by our increasingly complex multicultural environment. This impacts everyone from young and school-aged children with language acquisition and developmental issues to the elderly with neurogenic disease compounded by issues of bilingualism.

The academic pipeline is such that Hispanic students are not graduating in sufficient proportion to the general population so there is a dearth of Latin culture academic faculty in communication sciences and disorders. Carozza (2002) reported that there is a lack of resources in minority mentorship programs to successfully retain the young academic scholars who may be recruited through programs geared at earlier academic levels, such as programs geared toward college achievement. Internal mentorship is necessary for the successful senior Hispanic academics to reach down and support the talented scholars they may have trained. This is in keeping with the theme of this book to support speech-language pathology via mentorship at all levels of training from undergraduate, to graduate, to doctorate.

In today's world, there is a major reliance on electronic communication. Although there are strengths of online mentoring and supervision, there also are many gaps. In certain cultures it is the face-to-face and earnest interpersonal communication that is most highly valued. It is a challenge to both the multicultural supervisee as well as the multicultural supervisor to achieve the most efficient means by which to communicate about professional and personal career development. It also is a value to provide a role modeling dynamic in terms of professional demeanor. An online community will not be able to provide this. In some cases, we rely on a "virtual" supervisor, but possibly at a long-term cost. This can take the form of documents or clinic reports being edited by E-mail with bulleted "electronic comments" and no sense of explanation or origin of the comment. This may detract from the inspiration and creativity of supervision and dialogue. However, there are substantial reasons why "distance supervision" has come into vogue, not the least of which may be anticipated difficulty in dealing with a hard-to-supervise student clinician.

Nontraditional Students

Traditional supervision has been geared toward teaching American-born students whose culture is the same as the supervising environment. More recently, nontraditional students have entered the supervision arena, and supervising these students will encompass a whole new skill set. The nontraditional students may include the older returning student, the career changer, and/or individuals of varying cultural, social, and religious backgrounds, as well as sexual orientation. One of the contributions of this book is that it will put forth advances in the supervision of nontraditional students.

As reported by O'Callaghan, McAllister, and Wilson (2005), supervision has become increasingly complex in the United States and elsewhere, at both individual and institutional levels. The author describes that increased expectations have rendered certain supervisory practices as outmoded and, as such, actually may serve to impede clinical education. The same author compares United States models with standards of practice used in other countries. As an example, there is funding and innovative support to help stimulate innovations in programs in the United Kingdom. McAllister has continued to comment on what is like to be a clinical educator and the dilemmas they face: The dimensions that a good educator should encompass involve namely having a sense of self, a sense of relationship to others in the clinical environment, a sense of agency, and a desire to seek self-congruence and growth (Higgs & McAllister, 2007; Pappas, McLeod, McAllister, & McKinnon, 2008).

Multiple Dynamics

There currently exist several confounds in the literature primarily because each clinical scenario presents with its own unique factors. When the research pertains to actual clinical sessions, the ability to do research in supervision is complicated by the fact that each clinical triad (client-clinician-supervisor) is a distinct interpersonal dynamic that must be placed in objective terms to be evaluated scientifically. A contribution to the science of supervision involves a modification of the traditional scientific methodology that has come to be known as the gold standard in any evidence-based approach.

Reflection on Issues

As the case study scenarios throughout this chapter have illustrated, there is ample evidence that speech-language pathology is rapidly advancing as a profession. The opportunity to reflect on one's practice is perhaps the ultimate professional luxury. It is equally important to place one's profession in a socially relevant context. This renders growth, which is a critical element in life and work satisfaction.

Speech-language pathology has moved forward from the early years as a field of speech correction to one that embraces a tremendous array of clinical practice. From the neonatal intensive care units, to school-age literacy, to head and neck care in acute hospital settings, we are prepared for it all! It is inevitable as our world "shrinks" that the profession continues to strive to be as inclusive as possible. We have students, teachers, and clients from all over the world as a commonplace occurrence. Sensitivity to personal orientation is as equally significant as cultural awareness. This knowledge is one that helps us in personal development as well as in professional understanding. The issues related to all domains of cultural orientation will affect us, our clients, and other professionals.

It can be seen by this review of literature and case study research that the learning curve in the profession is remarkably steep, calling on skills that go beyond an expertise in the clinical speech and language behavior of our clients. This knowledge must stem from curriculum-directed initiatives that should be integrated in coursework and carried through professional education and the career of a speech-language pathologist. Matters of interpersonal differences obscure the clinical work at hand when we are dealing with the professional challenges of a diverse caseload. Sound practice calls for a rigorous and data-driven response to supervisory education. A place to begin can be training in self-reflection and application of a case study approach in a graduate ethics course. Self-analysis of clinical behavior also may assist in determining needs assessment and data collection. In this sense, we are focusing our clinical lens on ourselves as opposed to the client, while still using a problem-solving approach and the techniques that guide careful practice.

It is hoped that each reader will add to their own scope of practice by learning from previous models, gleaning information gained from the current literature, and perhaps establishing a rubric to guide a systematic method by which to supervise and potentially mentor other individuals both foreign-born and otherwise. Reviews of the literature should take into account differences in research methodology and factors related to the clinical nature of the discipline, which are compounded by global nature of the profession.

The main issues described in the challenges to supervision are centered around: cross-cultural differences, communication breakdowns, needs of nontraditional students, issues in clinical competence, and difficulty in application of classroom to real-world knowledge. The response to these issues is found in the gathering and sharing of individual knowledge. The knowledge of the self, on the part of the supervisor as well as the student clinician is critical if communication and trust are to be developed. The case studies have provided a point of reference and source of reflection as professional skills mature. Far-reaching insight can only be gathered painstakingly, and intimate knowledge and utilization of knowledge from all sources must be integrated to form a building source of supervisory wisdom. The next chapter brings forth recent information about current scientific approaches to supervision that shed important light on these

What's Next?

In the following chapter we look at some of the current approaches that may be used to address some of the issues described throughout this chapter.

Reflective Assignment

The reader is encouraged to reflect on the following questions as a means of beginning to think about the concepts introduced in this book:

- What do I know about supervision/mentoring?

- What do I want to know about supervision/mentoring?

- What do I feel are my strengths and weaknesses as a supervisor/mentor?

- What steps will I take to improve my knowledge and skills in these areas?

(Adapted from Zubizaretta, Campoy, & Ada, 2004).

CHAPTER 3

Current Approaches to Issues in Supervision Research

Be the change you want to see in the world.

Gandhi

Overview

A study of guided principles of supervision and its adaptations is increasingly critical given the complex challenges presented in the clinical arena. Therefore, it is important that supervisors do not take supervision as a given and endeavor to stay current with the latest practices and research trends. At the present time, the only requirement for becoming a supervisor is having obtained certification via completing coursework and clinical hours. However, there is no routine of formal training provided to prepare one for the role of a supervisor.

A survey conducted in 2008 by ASHA's Division 11 led to some interesting and revealing results on this very topic (see Appendix A). A total of 406 speech-language pathologists were surveyed with regards to their supervisory experiences and feelings about formal supervisory training. The majority of respondents were speech-language pathologists working in various settings whose supervisory experiences consisted primarily of graduate students and clinical fellows. A large majority of respondents indicted having received most of their supervisory training via self-study/readings (85%), on-the-job training (76%), and workshops/conferences (75%).

However, when asked about the importance of formal training, an overwhelming majority indicated a belief that formal training in supervision is very important (67%), particularly for new supervisors with no formal training and those who are seeking additional training.

Although such objectives are currently not underway, ASHA strives to address this need by providing information on the knowledge, skills, and necessary competencies of supervisors as well as the training standards for each level of clinical attainment (see references for a complete listing). Individual states also have their own guidelines and technical reports which outline the necessary competencies and may be provided by state agencies or external organizations (i.e., Joint Commission and Commission on Accreditation of Rehabilitation Facilities [CARF]).

In order to develop leadership skills and professional relationship models, we have to have knowledge in other areas of professional disposition. In the area of motivation and communication, there is less available and even less mandatory information taught on management styles and techniques. In recent research, clinical leaders are responding to the issues in supervision that face the profession.

The work of O'Connor (2006) in her article, "Supervision of Clinical Fellows: A Mentoring Process" is especially relevant. O'Connor's work is novel in that it speaks to the complexity of supervision. O'Connor herself describes that her supervisory experience started three years after graduate school when she became an "instant" supervisor. The author makes the point that clarifications of roles, expectations, and needs are essential to a successful experience. Planning carefully is also essential in making the expectations clear to everyone involved. She states that supervisees may gain insight via the process of seeing how their behaviors impact the clinical process and construct a hypothesis and examine it in terms of client response. Responsibility is placed on the supervisee to think about what strategies they have tried and become independent in modifying their behavior. The relationship becomes interdependent when the supervisor takes an indirect role in "unfolding" the supervisee.

Components of Supervision Training

In this article, O'Connor also outlines the five components of supervision, which are laid out in a series of stages as described in Table 3–1. These provide an ideal framework for the way in which supervision should be conducted, and lays out each of the areas that should be addressed in any supervisory dyad to ensure that the process runs smoothly. These guidelines were developed for use with clinical fellows, but also may be modified to use with supervisees at all levels of training.

O'Connor's (2006) work contributes to the important concept of team building based on mutual goals, open communication, and effective conflict resolution, and promotes an open outlook toward new challenges. More recently, O'Connor (2008) has raised further discussion regarding suggestions that could enhance supervision.

Table 3–1. Five Components of Supervision

Stage	Description
Stage I. Setting the Stage	• Provides information about supervisee's experience with certain populations and helps determine how much clinical instruction is needed
	• Expectations, goals, needs, re-evaluation, and analysis are defined and discussed
	• Involves gathering of pertinent information, including:
	Clinical Information
	1. General clinical experience
	2. Academic background
	3. Specific clinical experience with particular types of clients
	4. Clinical Fellow's perception of his or her own strengths and weaknesses
	5. Anxieties about working with clients who have _____ (disorder)

continues

Table 3–1. *continued*

Stage	Description
Stage I. continued	*Supervisee Information* 1. Type(s) of supervisory interaction experienced previously 2. Perception of self in terms of dependence/independence in general and with clients 3. Prior experience with data collection and analysis of client behavior 4. Experience with data collection and analysis of own clinical behavior 5. Perceptions of responsibility for bringing data and questions to the supervisory conference 6. Perceptions of assisting in problem solving, and decision making 7. Expectations for learning or modification of clinical skills from the current situation 8. Perception of need for feedback (amount and type)
Stage II. Training	• Teaching component of supervision • Supervisor responsibilities at this stage include: 1. Analyzing needs of the program, the clients, and the knowledge and skills of the supervisee 2. Determining how much demonstration (modeling) is necessary, how much practice is needed, and the best protocol to provide feedback to student 3. Taking the lead in demonstration and modeling of techniques
Stage III. Planning	• Planning for the client and the supervisory process, including: 1. Clinical activities 2. Observation 3. Data collection 4. Supervisory conferences 5. Self-analysis and evaluation

Table 3–1. *continued*

Stage	Description
Stage III. continued	• Supervisor is responsible for "operationalizing" the planning process and involving the supervisee at the level he/she is able to participate • Critical juncture in promoting independence of supervisee
Stage IV. Managing Schedules	• Managing and coordinating schedules, meeting times, and caseloads • Depending on environment, may include team meetings, class activities/schedules, etc. • May be useful to use electronic time management devices
Stage V. Evaluation	• Joint analysis of supervisee performance, including: *Formal Evaluation* • Use of standardized assessment tool such as the Clinical Fellowship Skills Inventory (see Appendix B for additional student/supervisor rating scales and assessment tools) *Informal Evaluation* • Periodic informal observations of supervisee are recommended • Supervisor and supervisee plan the objectives, format, and techniques they will use for follow-up discussions regarding intervention success • Supervisee should be informed of the format and techniques used for observation/ evaluation purposes • Recommended that supervisor use language that facilitates independent thinking and problem-solving by supervisee • Main objective is to increase capacity of supervisee for self-analysis • Should lead to the development of clear observations and relevant insights

Source: Adapted from O'Connor (2006)

She advocates for greater education about the supervisory process as well as increased documentation and research regarding the processes and tools that may assist in supervisory education and research.

One of the most interesting discussions raised about this topic was on the form of a recent online training seminar offered by http://www.speechpathology.com (Phillips & Sherman, 2009). The authors describe the continuity of the supervisory process. They state that supervision and mentorship may hark back to parenting experiences in terms of the success of interpersonal relationships. There are many challenges at several different levels. The student or the clinical fellow may not have been exposed to a variety of supervisory styles, and/or the supervisor may be working through the challenge of developing their own clinical style. They argue that even the term "clinical educator" has a different tone than "clinical supervisor."

They also note that different types of teaching or supervision are appropriate at different levels, whether the supervisee is an under-graduate, graduate student, clinical fellow, or fellow practitioner. Although there is a strong and necessary element of evaluation in standard supervisory practice about meeting basic competencies, good supervision involves a more cognitive approach to issues, including collaboration, self-knowledge, and the process of unfolding learning through shared experience. To paraphrase O'Connor (2006), supervisors should not mold, but rather seek to unfold their supervisees.

The notion that there can be a science of supervision and mentorship, therefore, is advanced by work such as this in that several concepts have been put forth by current practitioners who work in this area. They include: a study of guided principles of supervision is increasingly critical; a principled approach is necessary to establish standards of supervisory care; and that self-reflective learning done in a collaborative fashion is a starting point for the discoveries that will take place in the management of a communicatively impaired client.

This particular in-service raised several questions that need to be answered by the successful supervisor. A person who is supervised also deserves to have the knowledge of what their supervising has accomplished on the road to supervision. Therefore, it is important that all stakeholders share the power of knowledge in this relationship.

Basically, this raises the question, "On what basis is a supervisor supervising?" The same principle may be applied to other professional areas, even in allied areas such as management styles and techniques and leadership. Therefore, another principle involves the understanding of motivation. In the goals of developing leadership skills, and models of professional relationships, we have to have knowledge not only of the speech-pathology domain, but of other areas of professional disposition. In the area of motivation and communication, there is less available and even less mandatory information taught on management styles and techniques.

Another principle of guided practice in supervision is the understanding of not only client motivation, but also student and clinician motivation and how to engage in different communication modes to best suit different individuals and purposes. Management training in business offers one different communication techniques for different purposes such as presentation, persuasion, and explanation. Communication is enhanced when there is a sense of win-win, otherwise it arouses a state of conflict between the parties involved. This can affect the dynamics among the clinician, client, and/or supervisor. A consensus supervision style that calls for shared input and shared outcome is one that draws on these concepts. However, the practicalities of uneven levels of preparation by students and supervisors may not make this feasible.

Students and supervisors may be unfamiliar with the purpose and practice of this communication style, which is further compounded by cultural differences. The traditional as well as nontraditional supervisee/supervisor will have differing backgrounds and expectations that affect management of outcome. Contributing to this factor is the fact that in most settings there is a top-down communicative style due to administrative demands, which make these types of individual considerations difficult to maintain. However, a collaboration of communication styles drawing on all vested parties in the form of dialogue sessions, in addition to standard supervisory meetings, may help the supervisor and supervisee gain the mutual confidence and respect necessary for informed dialogue. In summary, informal dialogue is an essential component of management that serves to ensure that the motivation and commitment of all individuals is present. Please refer to Appendixes (C, D, E) for several examples of performance evaluation charts that can be completed by both the student and the supervisor to evaluate one another. These useful tools can act as a platform from which to begin a dialogue in order to ensure that all needs and expectations are being met. The KASA (found in Appendix F) can also be implemented for this purpose.

A supervisor must possess technical competence and finely honed skills in the management of resources, as well as human capital. Leadership skills may be modeled by learning from supervisory mentors to gain the administrative, interpersonal, and conceptual skills necessary for long-term success. A good supervisor and mentor is a socially perceptive and sophisticated individual who can perceive conflict before it begins and work to demonstrate how well-managed conflict can lead to growth. Scenarios such as role-play and case studies enable the new supervisor to delve into this domain prior to taking on supervisory responsibilities.

In summary, these aspects of developing a personal science of supervision emerge: the importance of a conceptual model, practice in utilizing the model, informal dialogue to know the stakeholder's interest and style, as well as especially fine skills in conflict mediation and negotiation. Based on some of the challenges noted as cited by the previous authors, additional responses to issues in supervision may involve greater education in motivational and management sciences. A novel suggestion for the profession would be an actual clinical supervisory practicum, which would be a setting in which a new supervisor would be able to practice his or her skills prior to taking on the role and responsibility of a supervisor. The ASHA Division 11 survey mentioned previously showed that a large percentage of professionals (86%) indicated willingness and likelihood to participate in such a course (see Appendix A). However, when asked what kind of training they were most likely to participate in, 96% of respondents cited online professional development conferences and workshops, as compared to a mere 40% who indicated willingness to take courses for credit. Not surprisingly, amount of time required and cost were the two most significant variables cited by respondents as the factors that would influence their decision to pursue such training. Refer to Appendix A for the complete results of this survey.

A supervisory mentor should be an individual who can help train supervisors on how to effectively deliver these skills and counsel supervisors on difficult situations. Ideally, this individual would possess years of experience as well as specific knowledge and competence of the research in supervision.

Future Directions for Supervision Training

One of the most important aspects of this developing communication style is the concept of true mutual respect. The use of objective feedback associated with the topic at hand and agreement between all parties is important in small and large problem-solving. This is a form of strategic supervision and should be practiced before any conflicts arise. There is a way of applying our clinical expertise as trainers to modeling an appropriate supervisor-supervisee relationship. Routine steps of a supervisory conference may assist in regulating and directing the supervisory conference. For example, in one group supervision conference workshop I have conducted, student clinicians are asked to discuss their cases in the form of a verbal acronym "SOAP." This terminology is well-known to practitioners and it basically applies to the notions of "S" standing for "subjective" case information, "O" for "objective" case information, "A" for "assessment" of progress within the session, and "P" for "planning" of future sessions. This practice greatly eliminated the type of case comments that do not further the training of the students. It also sharpened the thinking of the students regarding the issues at hand and gave them much needed verbal practice of putting their thoughts into concise words appropriate for professional meetings.

As supervisors and mentors, it is important to set the example and tone by requiring comments and routinely reviewing what students offer. The role of self-discipline is important in modeling consistency, responsibility for one's actions, and social reward for meaningful contributions in class. This will stimulate students to be independent problem-solvers who come prepared with solutions to clinical issues and are meaningful contributors to case planning. A strategy that emerged that can be incorporated into a measurement of effective supervision is that each clinician answers and responds to questions and contributes meaningfully. Each student has the opportunity for self-evaluation to express what they have learned about both their own and their client's performance. Aligned with this, students may have opportunities to develop comentoring skills by actively listening to, and providing feedback on, cases of their fellow students. In terms of my own practice, I have had success with students brainstorming solutions to case scenarios when they are taught how to listen as clinical peers. This was implemented in my courses in which I compared traditional top-down supervision models with peer-supervision models. Original student expectations were limited. However, final consensus was that the students stated that they learned more about their own case, as well as those of their peers, by acting as peer-supervisors.

In creating a model for evidence-based supervision, a review of studies has been provided in the form of a modified meta-analytic review of the literature. The next stage would be to compare the rigidity of scientific rigor applied to each study to determine what level of evidence has been achieved. Most of the studies are descriptive in nature. More work done in examining the same variables under controlled examination standards would allow for a test of empirical soundness as a model of standardization of care born from research. Researchers in supervision support the need for systematic research initiatives as per ASHA's technical report and recommend areas to be studied, including the effects on client outcome, which would be a critical element, as well as teaching effectiveness.

Furthermore, in related areas such as psychology, there is research that states that students who are mentored report more positive outcomes of their education as opposed to those who do not have mentors. A wealth of information appears in counseling literature regarding supervision, notably Fall and Sutton (2004). As a profession, speech-language pathology has contributed toward both supervision and mentorship as is discussed in detail in this book. It is perhaps difficult to apply the same scientific standards toward a goal of evidence-based mentorship. However, as all behavior can be measured by the right instrument, an attempt will be made to set forth some of the existing literature in this area, as well as a primary step in establishing a research base. The most effective supervision and mentorship methodologies should be goals of the speech-language pathology profession, as our profession depends heavily on the strengths of its supervisors and mentors.

It is of note that many related articles have begun to appear in the professional periodicals of the discipline, indicating that this topic is generating greater interest and more extensive research (Chabon, Hale, & Wark, 2008; O'Connor, 2008). Literature emphasizing team building and methodologies of best practice are especially prevalent (Ho & Whitehill, 2009; Shilpi & McAllister, 1999). One such example is Boone and Stech (1970), who reported on used self-confrontation and self-awareness strategies via videotaping and audiotaping of clinical speech sessions as a supervisory methodology to enhance clinical training.

Many researchers from disciplines external to speech-language pathology have approached this topic from different angles. Related to the work of Bandura (1997) is a study by Howard (2008). Howard's article stresses the use of positive psychology to enhance the effectiveness of clinical supervision. A sense of engagement is related to the clinician's and supervisor's well-being. Practitioners and supervisees can benefit from strategies that restore a sense of coherence. Specifically, the author mentions the use of narratives as a technique that may be applied successfully toward this end. Reflective practice is one of the meta-cognitive methodologies applied to the supervisory process within this book, which is echoed by others who study mentorship (Zubizaretta, Campoy, & Ada, 2004).

In the realm of general academe exists a body of research that attests to the academic success of students whose individual needs are considered during their training. Jacobi (1991) wrote about the importance of mentorship and effective undergraduate training, as did Juarez (1991). Nasim and Talley (2005) discussed the roles of race and gender in the politics of pedagogy in psychology. Thus, it is important that there exist a number of mentoring programs as a formal structure nationwide throughout different disciplines (National Education Association, 2005; National Mentoring Partnership [http://www.mentoring.org], 2010; Trautman, 2007).

One of the most engaging works I have read related to professional effectiveness is by Bandura (1997). The collection of research by this author points to the importance of self-efficacy. The work of Bandura (1997) has clear relevance to all educators. The importance of control over one's environment leads to greater confidence, as well as improved problem-solving. Hence, the perception of how much power one has in a given setting over decision-making, resources, instructional standards, parents, and community relate to the self-efficacy of teachers and clinicians, especially those in school-based settings. Therefore, included in this introduction is the effect of the environmental setting in how successful both a speech-language pathologist as well as his or her supervisor can become.

Under the lens of examination are the many factors that influence self-regulated learning. In an effort to provide an explanation of the behavior of the supervisor and supervisee, this book explores many factors that influence effort, persistence, and perseverance by both parties. Good clinical skills require a metacognitive awareness of oneself and others.

The concept of congruence repeatedly appears in the literature, as related to student satisfaction. To quote the work of Bordes and Arredondo (2005), "Students who perceived the environment as positive also reported higher levels of cultural congruity or having feelings of belonging" (p. 119). The notion of the cultural issues surrounding mentorship and supervision are examined extensively in this book. Many authors have reviewed scenarios thought to contribute to supportive learning communities. This is especially relevant in today's institutions of higher education with many students of diverse backgrounds. It is good practice to recognize the different characteristics of different learners. Programs such as the First

Fellows, described by Brommer and Eisen (2006), have attempted to address diversity from the standpoint of participation in the sciences from undergraduate to professoriate levels. A similar work by Gooden, Leary, and Childress (1994) discussed an initiative aimed at increasing engagement of minority faculty. This is especially timely in the field of communication sciences and disorders.

Another very relevant article was provided in the case study report by French (1997), who describes the task of supervising a speech pathology assistant, a category of paraprofessional recognized in some states. Professional supervision skills greatly impact service delivery and support the notion of preprofessional training in supervision in order for clinicians to function well in this responsibility area. At the 2006 ASHA National Convention, the "Supervision Boot Camp" addressed specific issues concerning the supervision of speech-language pathology assistants (SLPA) and provided reviews of the activities allowed for this group of employees, along with standards of supervision for the graduate intern, SLPA (Newman, O'Connor, Cabiale, & Victor, 2006). With this information in mind, it becomes evident that supervision can become a challenge for some. However, ASHA guides us in our need to supervise as long as we practice within an area of competence.

An experienced doctoral level speech-language pathologist trained as both a nurse and speech pathologist shared with the author her thoughts on the training differences in the two professions. In nursing, supervision standards were provided in the form of guides and checklists, whereas this was not the case when she entered speech pathology supervision. In fact, she stated that speech therapy practice itself appeared to differ widely from one clinician to another. She states that this is because communication is a system that depends on both participants:

> No matter how professional we are, we will never be robots who all do the same thing. Our personality is going to inform our therapy. So we are a little bit like psychologists in that regard. At the same time, we have goals that we want our clients to achieve, and that require certain actions on our part. (D. Ross, personal communication, September 2009)

The reader also is directed to Lubinski, Golper, and Frattali (2007) for a review of professional issues in speech-language pathology and audiology, which gives significant insight into the history of the professions and many underlying issues relevant to professional growth and longevity. With those thoughts in mind, the reader's attention will be drawn to issues of supervision and mentorship in a diverse society (Abesamis, 2007) and case study approach in addition to strategies gained through personal and professional experience in an effort to create a study of the principles of training.

This chapter explored some of the confounding issues in traditional supervision, advanced supervisory questions, and the challenges that we may encounter in trying to conduct research in this field. Some of the primary difficulties stem from the fact that objective measures are difficult to measure and analyze, as well as the fact that myriad factors play a role in the supervisor-supervisee relationship. We have looked at several case studies that highlight different issues and challenges that may arise. Differences in supervision at different training levels have been discussed. Thus, there are many important factors to keep in mind during this process.

What's Next?

It is up to the colleagues who read and respond to the themes of this book to extract from it what is new or reaffirming. This will contribute further to the goals of best supervision, best care, and best careers for all of us. On this note, contributions from practitioners are included in forthcoming chapters to analyze this topic from multiple, as well as shared, perspectives.

Reflective Assignment

CLINICAL COMPETENCIES	SELF-RATING		
	Very Competent	*Competent*	*Needs Work*
Ability to think conceptually and creatively.			
Ability to communicate effectively with individuals at different levels, including students and other professionals.			
Awareness of ethical and legal standards.			
Awareness of, and sensitivity to, multicultural issues.			
Sensitivity to supervisee's personal and professional development.			
Ability to both support and challenge supervisee.			
Ability to effectively collaborate with supervisee.			
Ability to maintain balance between the needs, goals, and objectives of both supervisee and client.			

CHAPTER 4

Multiple Perspectives Contributing to Supervision and Mentorship

The mediocre teacher tells. The good teacher explains. The superior teacher demonstrates. The great teacher inspires.

William Ward

Overview

This chapter continues the discussion of some of the issues inherent in clinical supervision and provides some expert opinions relating to supervision and mentorship. Included are key elements for developing self-awareness among professional individuals as our careers progress and as we become new supervisors. A contribution of this chapter is to recommend metacognitive approaches as an approach to the study of supervision. Metacognition refers to higher order thinking, which involves active control, over the active processes engaged in learning. Activities such as planning, how to approach a given learning task, monitoring comprehension, and evaluating progress toward completion of a task are metacognitive in nature (Livingston, 1997). As described below, these concepts can be applied to supervision.

Metacognitive Approach: Self-Supervision

The act of self-supervision is a form of a metacognitive task in that it involves reflection on our own tasks and behaviors. This may be an increasingly important construct because many clinicians are engaged as sole practitioners and are not actively supervised. Standards of practice are being evaluated and upgraded in the United States and elsewhere. McAllister (2005) has stated that increased expectations have rendered certain supervisory practices as outmoded, and as such, may actually serve to impede clinical education. McAllister also compares the United States models with standards of practice used in other countries. As an example, there is funding and innovative supports to help stimulate innovations in programs in the United Kingdom, whereas there is very little of such practice here in the United States.

McAllister has continued to comment on what is like to be a clinical educator and the dilemmas they face. The dimensions that a good educator should encompass involve having a sense of self, a sense of relationship to others in the clinical environment, a sense of agency, and a desire to seek self-congruence and growth (Higgs & McAllister, 2007; Pappas, McLeod, McAllister, & McKinnon, 2008).

In terms of the sense of agency, educators should seek to continuously evaluate themselves as they evaluate others. In keeping with this, McAllister (2005) conducted an analysis of supervision comparing traditional and peer supervision. In 2010, I conducted a self-evaluation contrasted with peer-group evaluation in the undergraduate clinic of an urban college in the form of a pre- and postassessment of expectations. The "ground" rules were determined by the group, and the end result was that the students expressed greater satisfaction in the outcome than they had anticipated. It was also shown that the students scored themselves lower than their peers had evaluated them. Although this project related to research presentations, this particular pattern has been described anecdotally in other instances in which everyone is their own harshest critic.

Introduction to Mentorship

What about mentorship? Is there really a science to it? Is there a difference between supervision and mentorship? The answer is a resounding "yes." Is there a science to successful supervision as it pertains to principled practice in types of cases in different diagnostic classes? The answer is also "yes." There is an expectancy that students share in their own self-education as they learn the intricacies of different disorders, their various representations, and evidence-based treatment protocols.

Is this different than mentorship? The answer is "yes." Is there a developing science to help guide the appropriate avenues and approaches to mentorship? That answer is also "yes." This answer can be seen through the activities of the American Speech-Language and Hearing Association (see ASHA Special Interest Division 11: Administration and Supervision, 2010d). Do individual clinicians have a responsibility to know the difference as they educate themselves on the roles they are taking on when they supervise or mentor newer clinicians? That answer is "yes." The focus of this book is to have a place to begin this dialogue, to read along with your mentee or mentor. Use this book in the curriculum so that expectancies are made mutually clear. This will enable us to better serve our clients and each other in the process.

Lisa O'Connor (2010) has discussed this topic in a recent Webinar regarding the learning focused approach to mentorship and supervision. A highly established and regarded colleague, O'Connor states that although lines can be "blurry," there are key differences between both practices. Supervision may include mentorship but not all mentorship includes supervision. There is not one essential continuum between the two. Central to the success of both is the criticality of communication. Throughout the literature, the need to define roles, responsibilities, and expectations is paramount, as is the need to "share" outcome expectations.

When issues develop in these processes, the experienced clinician must analyze where a possible lack of communication or miscommunication occurred. At the outset of any mentoring or supervisory relationship, the knowledge base of the junior clinician must be clearly realized. This is critical for effective management of appropriate outcomes and expectations. Salient criteria can be established in accordance to the needs of each setting. An important variable that relates to supervision and mentorship breakdown is emotional safety; learning takes place best in a climate of emotional safety. When we are dealing with supervisees or mentees of different cultures, ages, and/or generations, it takes special skill to generate the emotional safety that O'Connor describes. The many advanced aspects of supervision that are necessary to ensure these outcomes reinforce the notion that professional supervision is a distinct area of specialization to be considered in speech-language pathology training, and potentially certification.

There is an intimate interplay between the quality indicators of a good professional, whether they are a stand-alone practitioner, a supervisor, or a mentor. Accountability and adherence to practice models of a discipline is the hallmark of a professional. Special professionals possess the depth of earnestness, sensitivity, and compassion intermingled with broad professional expertise that allows them to be called on to mentor.

Who cannot remember a favorite teacher that they refer to as a mentor? This is at the heart of teaching, regardless of area of specialty. It is that moment that we decided this was our life's path. Frequently, it is accidental mentoring that takes place. Many times, the "mentor" is not aware of his elevated status in the eyes of the "protégé." We may not be officially apprenticing our student clinicians, yet there are qualities within specific teachers that resonate with specific students. This is very powerful and must be absorbed and accepted by both parties if it is to lead to a long-term relationship, which most do.

As this is inherently intangible, it is a goal of many researchers in mentorship to codify the behaviors and hence challenges of supervision. Therefore, the collection of information related to student attitudes and the associated perceptions of the supervisor is important to gauge routinely. Pre- and postresults may be obtained regarding not only how clients change, but also how clinicians change as a result of delivering therapeutic intervention. This is a function of reflective practice that can encourage a data-driven approach to the client's learning, as well as clinical growth.

In my own practice, I endeavor to make a study of the types of cases I have treated, their primary etiologies, the schedule of service, and length of service as a first step in personal leadership. The normative data one collects can help a sole practitioner or supervisor provide a new client with realistic outcomes and expectations at the point of referral. The acquisition of more uniform standards will enhance speech services provided to the most fragile members of society, children, and adults with disabilities, sometimes actually unable to speak for themselves. We do a disservice to students unless they start their careers with these standards (refer to ASHA for the complete listing) in mind. To develop this notion in young professionals, it is important to expose them systematically to quality indicators of research. The integration of the unique aspects of each case and each clinician also should be acknowledged.

At the 2006 meeting of the regional conference of the National Aphasia Association in New York City, a movement was launched called a "Patient's Bill of Rights for Aphasics." This notion is important for the many clients and families that lack a full understanding of the professional training of clinicians and the duty-bound aspects of a profession. This particular proposal was met with great enthusiasm because in the controlled hospital setting, patients who have language loss may not get access to their own medical information in a format they can understand. Hospitals provide translators for foreign language speakers, Braille for the visually impaired, and sign language interpreters for hearing impaired. However, there is no uniform standard for language adjustments to accommodate those with aphasia.

In every population, the need for clear and principled supervision, be it by outside parties or self-supervision, is integral to providing a sound product of service delivery that can stand up to the scrutiny of outside professionals. Vision cannot be taught, but leadership principles can.

Views on Supervision and Mentorship

Another important consideration is that students and professionals at all levels, whether they be undergraduate, graduate, CFY, or certified clinicians already involved in a professional life, should be concerned about what their work arena will consist of in terms of structure and leadership. If we know what to expect in a good supervisory relationship, there is better opportunity for fruitful engagement. Therefore, there is something to be gained in establishing meaningful benchmarks for all readers in terms of the concepts of supervision and how they may be applied in different settings in an effort to develop a science of supervision that can be adaptable to many levels of interaction.

Metacognitive Approaches to Supervision

The need for a solution generated by a problem is more complex than a linear equation of one problem–one solution. A careful practitioner and his or her supervisor closely examine the root causes. However, there generally are multiple interacting causes that complicate the resolution. Analysis of the maintaining factors also is crucial. Many times a situation is perceived as less than perfect but is relatively acceptable and therefore is maintained by the "status quo." Lack of concerned service delivery may permeate some disciplines, but speech-language pathology is one field in which this cannot be interjected. First, we are primarily dealing with children and their educational welfare and this translates into everyone's concern. Second, the field has established broad and respected governance in the form of our certifying national body, ASHA. It is on the foundation of this concerted leadership that most of our careers are built and equally sustained. Therefore, a multirooted situation requires a multiple level response that has visible and lasting benefits to those who seek improved supervision.

Quality Assurance

It is the ethical responsibility of speech-language pathologists and their supervisors to provide quality care. The success of sound supervision can be established through the use of quality assurance studies. A quality assurance network is one way in which concerned clinical supervisors can establish benchmarks for points of excellence such as client outcomes, satisfaction, and effectiveness.

One such survey was done by the author during the development of a new teaching clinic program. Items were divided into five categories: benefit, courtesy, preparedness, efficiency, and comfort. The benefit of such a survey is that examples of each category can be customized to various settings. Perceptions can be rated on a linear scale and compared across time and/or observers for consistency and change.

Examples:

Benefit: I am "better" because I received these services.

Courtesy: Staff was courteous and pleasant.

Preparedness: Clinician was prepared and organized.

Efficiency: Length and frequency of program was appropriate.

Comfort: Health and safety precautions were taken.

Gordon-Pershey and Reese (2002) also report on consumer satisfaction surveys as a means by which to measure quality assurance. Gordon-Pershey and Reese (2002) state that such measures may be beneficial not only for the improvement of clinical services, but also may be directly applied during supervision as a means by which to further students' development of clinical skills. Anderson (1988, as cited in Gordon-Pershey and Reese, 2002) reported that a poll of the supervisory needs of speech-language pathology students revealed that they wanted their supervisors to coach them in becoming procedure-oriented and in providing feedback to clients. Consumer survey data can provide information about areas where students feel less secure, such as to assess whether particular procedures were successful or whether feedback to clients was sufficient.

Opportunity for patient and peer feedback is critical in self-supervision. The ability to work side by side with other seasoned clinicians is a form of "checks and balances" for clinical directors and supervisors. The supervisor serving as the sole senior practitioner must create new forms of feedback from outside parties. The application of this model and ones like it are derived from the business management practices of accountability for product marketing, delivering, and repairing. These same tenets were brought up in an interview with John F. Robinson, President and CEO of the National Minority Business Council, a premier business development organization serving the nonprofit sector. A responsibility to ensure consistency of goods through the business cycle can also apply to the delivery of services. As of yet, though, there has been no such model for delivery of supervisory services.

There is a huge concentration of the successful delivery of services to clients based on etiology, but who is "watching" the supervisor? If we believe in the top-down model, the ethics and strategies of the supervisor should trickle down just as much as the clinical educational material. It is the protection of the continuum of care that makes a vision for excellence in leadership so important, especially with the increasing challenges in the 21st century. Public accountability is all around us. The combination of both internal and external monitoring is crucial to sustain good practice.

It may be surprising for new clinicians to understand the liability and obligation they have when they take on a case, diagnose, and offer remediation. "Lack of outcome" is a new concept that I believe will enter the field sooner rather than later. One attempt made to respond to this issue has been proposed by The National Outcomes Measurement Survey (NOMS) project of ASHA, which is among several organizations that attempts to quantify outcomes for purposes of quality assurance. The primary models come from medicine. An entire specialty of nursing is devoted to "Quality Assurance" and the risk management arena.

Risk management is important to use in speech pathology in that we are responsible for the services we deliver. We must be informed about potential treatment outcomes, our approach of choice, and rationale for choosing one strategy over the other. This is only one aspect of quality assurance in the field. Others may be accountability to peers, subordinates, and management as well as the typical end of the year client satisfaction surveys popular in some settings.

A problem with this approach is that the respondents tend to be public consumers who do not have the same level of information as the provider. Therefore, effectiveness cannot be solidly measured. It is the review by external peers and comparison with industry-wide standards that speech-language pathology must face. Because it still is a relatively young profession, the benchmarks are just being established. However, there are millions of adults and children counting on the fact that their clinician and supervisory team are delivering the best possible treatment for their disorder.

In many cases, the speech-language pathologist serves as their own supervisor, especially after receiving their certification from ASHA. Is the answer that we self-monitor our own work? In remote areas or in underserved populations, self-monitoring may have to be the solution. Just as we have mandatory continuing education to maintain licensure, it is should be necessary to track one's own quality. A vision for leadership can be borrowed from medical communities regarding how incidents are tracked. Implications for change may be made based on the response to the incident. Setting up preventive programs potentially will cut down on incidents of a similar nature. Such vision is a hallmark of leadership—it is what separates managers from leaders.

In an independent survey conducted by the present author for purposes of obtaining perspectives from current in-the-trenches supervisors from multicultural backgrounds, the following top 10 characteristics were identified by the group as being essential to a satisfactory supervisory dyad. They are:

1. Communication.

2. Mutual expectations from the curriculum.

3. Shared knowledge of classroom models.

4. Subordinate structures for discussion of special issues.

5. Strong clinical knowledge of population to be serviced.

6. Strong educational preparation of the student clinician in techniques of childhood education in the case of pediatric placements.

7. Accessibility of supervisory input.

8. Mutual civility.

9. A strategy for quick assistance on as-needed circumstances.

10. Consideration for the totality of the personal as well as the professional growth of the student clinician.

To follow up on this, original questions were developed for response by clinical educators (Table 4–1).

In this chapter we introduced the concept of mentorship, and examined some of the differences between mentorship and supervision. We looked at some newer approaches to thinking about supervision. Last, this chapter addressed issues of quality assurance, both to our clients as well as to our supervisees.

What's Next?

In the following chapter, issues of accountability are addressed further with a discussion about the code of ethics and how this guides both our clinical practice and our role as supervisors and mentors.

Reflective Assignment

Think about a clinical supervisor and/or mentor who had a significant influence on your life. In what ways did this person contribute to your personal and/or professional development? What strategies or techniques did they employ that you found beneficial? Think about their style of interaction and communication, the kind of information that was shared, how personal or sensitive thoughts and feelings were addressed, and so on. What did you admire most about him or her and in what ways can you strive to adopt some of those qualities in your own practice?

Table 4–1. Needs Analysis Survey for SLP Supervisors

	Strongly Disagree 1	Mildly Disagree 2	No Opinion 3	Mildly Agree 4	Strongly Agree 5
1. Do you believe there could be greater science used in supervision (i.e., data-based practices)?					
2. Do you believe that SLP supervision is objective?					
3. Do you believe there is too much subjectivity in supervision?					
4. In thinking back over earlier supervision you have done, would your present experience change any prior student assessments?					
5. Do you believe that supervision and/or mentorship can be quantified?					
6. Do you have self-standards of supervision that you apply in a uniform fashion to all your supervisees?					
7. Do you believe that supervision training should be mandatory?					

continues

Table 4–1. *continued*

	Strongly Disagree 1	Mildly Disagree 2	No Opinion 3	Mildly Agree 4	Strongly Agree 5
8. Do you believe that you had adequate training as a supervisor when you first entered supervision?					
9. Do you feel that speech-language pathology supervision should be specialized/and or board-certified?					
10. Do you believe that more evidence-based supervision research is necessary?					
11. Do you use a standard/formal operational definition that separates supervision and mentorship?					
12. Do you believe that outcome measures are needed in supervision and mentorship?					
13. Do you do a self-assessment of your competencies in supervision?					
14. Have you ever turned down opportunities to supervise?					
15. Do you consider supervision as professionally superior to direct service?					

	Strongly Disagree 1	Mildly Disagree 2	No Opinion 3	Mildly Agree 4	Strongly Agree 5
16. Do you believe every speech-language pathologist should be equipped to be a supervisor upon certification?					
17. Do you think that a supervision certification would be a good idea for the field of speech-language pathology?					
18. Have you had positive supervision experiences throughout your career?					
19. Using your own definitions, do you believe every speech-language pathologist is qualified to be a mentor?					
20. Do you actively participate in ASHA special interest division activities on mentorship?					
21. Do you receive sufficient mentorship for yourself in your supervisory activities?					
22. Is your primary professional identity a supervisor as opposed to as a clinician?					

continues

Table 4–1. *continued*

	Strongly Disagree 1	Mildly Disagree 2	No Opinion 3	Mildly Agree 4	Strongly Agree 5
23. Do you believe that learner outcomes can be established for prospective supervisors?					
24. Would you agree with mandatory continuing education in supervision and mentorship?					
25. Do you believe that supervision and mentorship models should be updated to include nontraditional students and global learners?					

CHAPTER 5

Ethical Considerations in Supervision and Mentorship

We can teach from our experience, but we cannot teach experience.

Sasha Azevedo

Introduction to Ethics

Thus far, this book has explored the current status of supervision, relevant issues and challenges, responses to these issues, as well as strategies for dealing with these issues. As a lifelong practitioner, the scientific underpinnings applied in my research and practice as a clinician and a supervisor have been described. Case study scenarios have been provided as examples to illustrate some of the challenges described. A cumulative discussion of the competencies and strategies are described in the subsequent chapter. Now we get into the ethical responsibilities of supervision.

From a practical standpoint, the policies and procedures, in addition to the scope of practice, are contained within the ASHA documents and are covered in graduate education as well. However, the way in which to become an exemplary clinician and supervisor ultimately is up to the individual. Initially, in an effort to protect all individuals involved, it is important to establish limitations of practice in each setting in terms of what is required by the staff, the supervisor, and other parties. Issues of ethics and liabilities emerge and should be dealt with from a priority basis prior to service delivery. This may include policies and procedures and contracts as well as in-service orientation to items such as risk prevention, accidents, incidents, and infection control. These parameters should be evaluated on an ongoing basis.

The challenges we face in our daily personal lives have increased exponentially. Similarly, the complexities of working within an allied health profession have increased tremendously as well. If we are to have long and productive careers, supervisors must anticipate and be prepared to handle individual differences, multicultural issues, and higher public expectations. Imagine a new clinician who is more knowledgeable about a technical service delivery than the supervisor is. These situations abound especially in medical speech pathology, a growing subspecialty in the field.

The security of the client, the new clinician, and the supervisor may be jeopardized if the supervisor's knowledge base does not extend into specific areas of subspecialization. This can take place despite the best intentions of the treatment team. There simply are too many areas of specialization to make a good match for every supervisee-supervisor dyad.

Who then should assume this burden? One place to which we may look for guidance on such important matters of professional development is ASHA, our national governing organization. The leadership of ASHA provides the professional body with the essential resources and guidelines necessary for establishing clinical practice (Lubinski & Frattali, 2000). In our role as supervisors we must challenge and empower ourselves to look beyond the core requirements of licensure in order to take on the responsibility of mentoring a new clinician. In effect, we are bridging the gap between the client and the student who will be working with that particular client in the future. Thus, in essence we are doing double duty by taking on the responsibility for both the personal growth of the client, as well as the personal and professional growth of the student. This may be in a number of varied settings, including schools, college clinics, hospitals, and nursing homes.

It is a daunting task to say that in the nine months of a clinical fellowship year, a clinician can prepare for a life of work. Therefore, concerned professionals continue to further their education and to seek further support and learning through various clinical activities, journal reading, and seminar attendance. However, the type of independence that an internalized vision can provide transcends the learning of new theory. It is to make one's own model or "vision for leadership." These values can follow a clinician through new territories as we change settings, geographic location, or re-enter the workplace, all of which are now quite commonplace. A "one-size-fits-all" model for supervising others or oneself is no longer suitable.

The supervisor who takes on the responsibility and presents him or herself as qualified to teach and supervise others actually assumes the burden of care to the patient and responsibility to their supervisee. The supervisor must seek out quality education and materials about the cases under their charge, in addition to seeking out information regarding their new roles and responsibilities. In order to address such issues of professionalism and accountability, ASHA (2010) has issued a Code of Ethics policy statement (Appendix G). The Code of Ethics policy statement clearly delineates all of the legal, ethical, and moral codes that professionals in the discipline must adhere to in order to provide the most effective and appropriate services to clients and families.

Among the roles and responsibilities outlined in this document, some of the most significant ones include the responsibility to represent ones' self fairly and accurately (i.e., citing appropriate credentials, training, education, experience); to effectively evaluate the quality and provision of services rendered; to engage only in those aspects of the profession that are within one's scope of practice; to adequately inform clients about all potential risks and benefits of intervention; to provide accurate, evidence-based research to support claims regarding nature and management of communication disorders, professional issues, and research/scholarly activities; to not discriminate against peers, students, and colleagues in allied professions regardless of age, gender, ethnicity, religion, sexual orientation, disability, and so forth, as well as to adhere to principles of confidentiality with regard to client information and provision of services rendered (see Appendix G).

In practice, SLP's are allowed to practice all activities for which they are clinically competent. However, it is an ethical dilemma in some cases to substantiate requisite experience when applying for a new position. One example can be seen in a current situation in which a facility sought to protect itself from licensed, but less experienced, hires. The facility ran an employment advertisement that called for documentation of a specific number of hours performing the modified barium swallow (sophisticated instrumentation used for clients with suspected swallowing and feeding issues that requires extensive training). SLPs frequently are hired based on a resume, recommendation letters, and a strong interview rather than number of documented hours of training in a particular technique under a licensed supervisor. If this is not the case, an agency may opt to provide hands-on training at the cost of the institution. This may be exacerbated with a shortage of qualified practitioners currently practicing, especially in certain areas of the field.

It caught my attention because SLP's are interpreting whether they have sufficient experience to take on a certain task. What is considered "sufficient" is not always clear, even in medically challenging environments. This calls on the ethics of the hiring agency to ensure that the competencies of the hired individual are sufficient; as well as the site supervisor charged with overseeing patient care.

In addition to the shortage of clinicians, there also is a shortage of clinical supervisors. How then do we effectively and appropriately deal with such issues of professional accountability and subsequently adhere to the Code of Ethics? In some cases, CF's must find their own supervisors based on a fee, thus treating supervision as an outsourced business. In some cases, facilities may opt to assume the burden for inexperienced clinicians by taking on a facility malpractice policy. Malpractice policies presumably protect patients and practitioners, which is why hospitals and other challenging environments will only accept graduate students with relevant coursework for externships. However, it may be difficult to obtain such a position for a student even with the necessary background coursework. In all instances, no facility or professional wants to put themselves at legal risk because even if not proved factual, it is enough to potentially ruin a career. In extreme cases, these professionals may be censured, lose certification, and lose licensure.

Different skill sets are the growing trend in the field of speech-language pathology. The generalists of yesteryear will find themselves frustrated and without a clear scope of practice. However, this does not mean that they then should supervise! After years of dedicated direct service, supervisors return to "train others." The quality of training is put at risk unless the supervisor has studied how to supervise with the same vigor and intensity as he or she studied the elements of speech-language pathology as a discipline.

Introspection and the support of fellow supervisors serve to identify risk within the field and its practitioners. As the old adage goes, no one person can know everything. A responsible professional must know their strengths and weaknesses and seek to apply themselves to developing a personal path for growth. In the preceding chapters, we have examined the importance of common goals in supervision. Shared expectations, personal qualities, and communication styles underlie a professional and scientific approach to supervision. Applied to oneself, these principles can form a framework for an individual leadership guide. Case studies, vignettes, focus groups, and informative interviews are other avenues by which a sole practitioner seeking to further develop their supervisory style can become better informed. In addition to the educational and professional challenges of being a supervisor, there are significant legal and ethical responsibilities as well.

This chapter provided an in-depth discussion of ASHA's Code of Ethics and how these guidelines impact our practice as clinicians and as supervisors. As health care practitioners, it is our responsibility to adhere to these guidelines and provide the best and most effective possible services.

What's Next?

This completes the first part of the book relative to understanding the issues surrounding supervision and mentorship from my perspective, including major history, operative definitions, and issues bearing on accountability, good practice, and challenges. In the subsequent chapters, the discussion continues with a review of research strategies, as well as professional competencies drawn from multiple perspectives. Questions for further study and contributions to the area of successful supervision and mentorship in speech-language pathology are described.

Reflective Assignment

Read the following case scenarios below (Morehouse, Rodgers, & Waguespack, 2006) and think about whether or not each of these violates the Code of Ethics (see Appendix G). If so, which principle do they violate? How would you handle each situation?

Case Scenario #1

A Fort Lauderdale SLP who is planning to get married over the weekend and go on her honeymoon the following week is intent on having all paperwork completed before she leaves work on Friday. On Thursday, she completes the Medicaid billing for the month and includes therapy sessions for two children who are usually seen on Friday mornings. The therapy logs indicate that both children are absent on Friday, but she submits the billing as it was completed with the intention to omit one of the Medicaid billings for the next session with the children. After an audit, a complaint is filed by Medicaid officials.

Case Scenario #2

An SLP assistant working with a client with ADHD and a language impairment complains to her supervisor because she feels she needs help in dealing with the student's significant behavioral problems as well as the language disorder. She feels she is not getting enough supervision but the supervisor states that she's too busy to give more time to the assistant. The supervisor tells her she already should have learned in her coursework what to do with clients like this. The assistant voices her concerns to the department head who then files a formal complaint.

Case Scenario #3

An SLP dismisses a client from therapy after repeatedly discouraging his sexual advances. She provides him with a referral list of three SLPs. The client reviews the list and tells her which SLP he has selected but refuses to sign a release of information. Concerned that a colleague may be subjected to the same sexual advances, she calls her colleague to warn her of this client's behavior.

SECTION II

Developing Knowledge and Skills as a Supervisor and Mentor

CHAPTER 6

Supervisory Competencies and Strategies

*The teacher who is indeed wise does not bid you
to enter the house of his wisdom but rather leads
you to the threshold of your mind.*

Kahlil Gibran

Overview

This chapter is divided into two sections. The first section focuses on several of the competencies necessary to be an effective supervisor, which include an understanding of interpersonal communication styles, cultural and linguistic factors, personal resilience, and sensitivity to social power. The second section focuses on specific strategies designed to increase effectiveness of supervision using current research trends. These include conversational analysis, reflective practice, and personal narratives.

This chapter also describes the dynamics of supervision, some of which have not been extensively applied to speech-pathology supervision in an integrated manner, as they have been in other disciplines. Some of the constructs discussed are presented as an outgrowth of my professional experience in an effort to shed further light on competencies and strategies that have served me in my career. As such, it is felt that a strong basis in essential foundations from ASHA, coupled with new applications of information, are highly useful.

Barrow and Domingo (1997) assert that clinical supervisors receive little if any preparation for their role as supervisors. We can train interactions; however, there is a distinction between direct and indirect supervisory styles. As each individual supervisee develops, they will be more personally proactive in terms of their development. The goal of the supervisor is to establish an independent professional and the goal of the clinician to achieve that independence. In the most common supervision scenario, the CF year, ASHA provides leadership on the conduct of the supervisor and the requisite underlying abilities (ASHA, 2010e).

During the clinical fellowship year, the supervisor is referred to by ASHA as the mentor of the clinical fellow. Their chief role is to provide meaningful mentoring and feedback as well as assist the clinical fellow in developing independence. The minimum mentoring requirements are 6 hours of direct supervision per each 3-month segment and six indirect monitoring activities per segment. These may include review and evaluation of treatment plans and target goals, as well as monitoring the clinical fellow in professional meetings and other collaborations. The competencies outlined in this chapter would provide a good baseline for a more sensitive clinical supervisory process that would optimize the training of professional delivery of services.

The new supervisor, in supervising his or her first clinical fellow, will utilize the lead instrument, which is the Clinical Fellowship Skills Inventory (CFSI) developed by ASHA (see Appendix B). This contains a description of each skill and a rating system. The CFSI is a rating scale consisting of a set of 18 skills involved in the four areas of evaluation, treatment, management, and interaction. It is conducted at least once during each of the three segments of the clinical fellowship year. It can be found at http://www.asha.org/ce rtification/Clinical-Fellowship.

The ability to supervise and mentor another individual can be a very fruitful career path. In their quest for self-knowledge McCready and Raleigh (2009) encourage supervisors to reflect on their own attitudes toward people and their worth, be honest about the values they bring to the supervisory process, understand their own perceptions of their role, analyze the rationales for their own behavior, and determine if their behaviors are consistent with their basic philosophy of supervision.

Successful supervision and mentorship go hand in hand and the longevity of a speech-language pathologist can be enhanced by the knowledge of effective supervision. We can teach our incumbent supervisees more confidently armed with evidence. One of the most significant findings of Owen and colleagues, from the psychology discipline, was that mentorship led to increased personal satisfaction and improved performance (Owen & Solomon, 2006; Owen, Solomon, Mallozzi, Kline, & Wareham, 2007a, 2007b).

Supervisory effectiveness requires not only an in-depth understanding of the various disorders and possible treatment options, but also an understanding and appreciation of both the technical competencies and useful strategies which may enhance supervision. From the standpoint of a clinical interaction, it would be considered ethically wrong for a clinician to treat a case in which they have little knowledge and experience. In order to obtain this knowledge, we thus must seek out specific training and educate ourselves to provide the best possible service to our clients.

Competencies

The competencies necessary to be a skilled supervisor include an understanding of interpersonal communication styles, cultural and linguistic factors, personal resilience, and sensitivity to "social power" (Wagner & Hess, 1997). For illustrative purposes, the competencies necessary for supervision are exemplified through feedback from real-life supervisory dialogues. It should be noted, however, that each of these competencies has its own nuances that should be explored and further researched. As such, one example of a tool that may be used to increase one's awareness of these issues is the Multicultural Developmental Supervisory Model (MDSM), established in psychology (Field, Chavez-Korell, & Domenech Rodriguez, 2010). This model integrates specific Latina/o multicultural counseling competencies and Latina/o ethnic identity theory with developmental theories of supervision. It is designed to identify the complex processes that influence the supervisory dyad in an effort to provide guidance and support to the supervisor and the supervisee, as well as the institutions in which supervision takes place.

Interpersonal Communication Styles

All professional fields stress the importance of interpersonal communication skills as a key aspect. According to O'Connor (2008),
most people view communication skills as an innate human ability
or something that is learned through trial and error. However, this
is not always the case. Individuals may not always be aware of how
they come across to others and their conversational styles. If individuals have very different styles of communicating, due to cultural,
linguistic, and/or other factors, this in essence may impact the
effectiveness of their dialogue. Such issues are especially relevant
during supervisory conferences, when the student and supervisor
are engaged in a dialogue pertaining to the clinical work.

According to Clinical Supervision in Speech-Language Pathology, put forth by ASHA (2008a), aspects of interpersonal communication reported to be most highly regarded included unconditional
positive regard, earnestness, empathy, and concreteness. McCrea
and Brasseur (2003) also noted that effective communication style
was shown to have a positive effect on the supervisee's willingness
to interact and participate, and hence positively affect the supervisory relationship.

Enhancing clinicians' sensitivity to their own conversational
styles can also be beneficial because, as clinicians, we must deal
with a great many people in our professional lives. And because all
of these individuals undoubtedly exhibit very different personali-
ties and conversational styles, it would only serve to benefit us to
be able to adapt our own conversational styles to those with whom
we must interact on a daily basis as professionals. The following are
examples, using the tool of metapragmatic assessment:

> Supervisor: I can't believe that I said, "you know" that many
> times. I know that, you know, it's so like typically female but
> I really just can't believe that I said it that many times. And
> "um" too; "like" as well. And I'm kind of a stutterer as well.
>
> Student: I kind of feel like that it sounded as if I was aware
> of the recording. I don't know so much about that or maybe

that's the way I normally speak and I never realized that before. But I try my best to think things through but then, and then I find that I'm really verbose. Um, I say "um" a lot. I always think that I'm the type of person to cut people off before they finish and, um, finish off phrases for them without giving them a chance to finish so I was glad to hear that I gave her a chance to speak.

Cultural/Linguistic Factors

There currently exist a number of training programs for cultural and linguistic competencies among the helping professions, including groups such as physicians. Completion of "mandated" competencies is not enough in today's world. It takes personal commitment and self-reflective practice to carry through the goals of informed supervision. A thoughtful practice of journal-keeping is one model by which a mature clinician can guide their own journey to awareness, as described by McCready and Raleigh in their article, "Creating a Philosophy of Supervision Through Personal Narratives" (2009). This practice will help to increase personal sensitivity toward the clients we treat and the student clinicians we supervise. The following case scenario illustrates how cross-cultural differences bridged between supervisor and student indicate that differences in styles enhance the establishment of rapport.

> Supervisor: I have a tendency to talk fast. I don't know if it's because I've lived in New York all my life but I'm sure. I feel like we have a good conversation. We've had some really nice conversations about how life is like in Trinidad [the student's birthplace] and I think that the way she talks is definitely cultural.

> Student: We had good, you know, communication. She's, um, getting to know me better and I'm getting to know her and we accept each other. You know, she accepts me and my personality and background and I accept her.

Personal Resilience

Salvatore Maddi (2005) contributed to the literature by developing the Hardiness Survey. The ability to learn from one's own professional life and experiences contributes to one's own problem-solving abilities, which in turn can be imparted to others. Inevitably, work settings will be met with conflicts that may challenge even the most experienced supervisor. The constructs of self-discipline and "hardiness" will help the supervisor deal effectively with the subordinates, staff, and so forth. Conflict resolution, stress management, and coping styles are all interpersonal skills that a mature supervisor should possess. Interested readers may complete this survey online via the Hardiness Institute (see references).

In other disciplines such as psychology, it is necessary to receive supervision and therapeutic support throughout one's professional career. However, although this currently is not the adopted practice in speech pathology, it bears consideration. This is because, inevitably, a long career will be impacted by personal and/or professional challenges at various points in time. Astute supervisors will seek outside support in the form of self-knowledge to help them sustain a high level of practice and maintain professionalism. The work of Maddi (2005) is but one of many examples in which insight into this complex area may be gained.

Social Power

Power has been defined as "the ability of one party to change or control the behavior, attitudes, opinions, objectives, needs, and values of another party" (Rahim, 1989, p. 545). According to Bass (1981, as cited in Wagner & Hess, 1997), social power has an integral role in the supervisory process. It serves as a form of influence with trainees so that they effectively change their clinical behaviors. Social power has been measured via psychometric inventories such as the Rahim Leader Power Inventory (RLPI) in various industries worldwide (as cited by Wagner & Hess, 1997).

Real power should come from real skills and preparation to do the job so that staff can have honest respect for their leadership and minimize any conflicts that may arise from discrepant perceptions of social power in the work setting.

Outcome measures are better managed when perceptions are aligned at the outset of a supervision encounter. A formal way to do this may be to administer instruments such as a modified RLPI (Wagner & Hess, 1997) or the Powell Attitude Survey (1987) to the staff and supervisors at significant junctures within the clinical process. This would be a way in which to acknowledge the impact of perception and power as well as expectations. An additional consideration may be to develop one's own outcome assessment measure using several foundation questions such as: *What is supervision? What do I expect to gain from this supervisory experience? What type of supervision am I most comfortable providing/receiving? What should students and supervisors expect from each other?* (adapted from Manderson, 1997). This can be done in either a written or verbal format and may be a good way to begin the first supervisory meeting with a new supervisee. It would enable both student and supervisor to gauge a comparison of perceived outcomes and expectations. It may help to start a discussion about these issues, and has the potential for long-term benefit of the supervisor/mentor relationship.

Training in Supervisory Competencies

The Administration and Supervision Special Interest Division of ASHA provides leadership to the profession in the area of supervision, with a scope that goes beyond the purpose of this book. New and continuing supervisors are urged to avail themselves of their publications, newsletters, and presentations. One of the many great contributions to the study of supervision was written by Shelly Victor (2001) in which she describes the elements of establishing coursework in supervision.

In this work, Victor (2001) provides an essential contrast between the master's level training that may include a course in supervision and those doctoral programs that include a required course in supervision, which is becoming increasingly more prevalent in clinical doctoral programs such as the SLP.D degree. The issue is that while many Ph.D. and Ed.D. degree holders have supervisory or administrative functions, they have never had a course in how to train or supervise clinical functions. For these reasons, the contrasts between the two levels of preparation are important to include in a chapter on supervision and mentorship. Victor (2001) makes the important distinction that:

1. Master's students **have the option** to take a course in supervision.

2. Doctoral students are **required** to take a course in supervision.

The course outcomes in Table 6–1 are gleaned from Victor's article.

Victor (2001) also provides a summary of the course objectives that would be useful in planning for supervisory training platforms:

- Components of supervision and the supervisory continuum

- Roles of the supervisor and supervisee

- Styles of supervision

- ASHA's 13 supervision tasks

- Data collection techniques

- Roles of the supervisee and supervisor during the supervisory conference

- Supervisor and supervisee assessment tools

- Legal and ethical issues in supervision

- Facilitating communication and resolving conflicts

- Supervision across settings

- Professional requirements for supervision

Table 6–1. Comparison Between Masters and Doctoral Levels of Study

Masters Level	Doctoral Level
1. Discuss components of the supervisory process.	1. Discuss the contribution and influence made by many of the classic studies in the field of supervision.
2. Utilize the ASHA 13 competencies in supervisory planning.	2. Plan the supervisory conference for the client, clinician, supervisor, and supervisee.
3. Describe supervisory continuum.	3. **Utilize a variety of data collection systems to observe the supervisory process.**
4. Discuss various styles of supervision.	4. Analyze the data obtained during the supervisory process
5. **Utilize a variety of data collection systems to observe the supervisory process.**	5. Integrate the results of the data analysis to the goals within the context of the supervisory conference.
6. Plan a supervisory conference.	6. Establish a framework for a personal style of supervision.
7. Discuss current issues in supervision.	7. Discuss and integrate current research findings in the field of supervision.
8. Develop a plan for self-supervision.	

At the Master's level, the students appear to be taught how to discuss procedures and have limited freedom to provide hands-on experience. Master's level students develop knowledge on how to provide adequate "self-supervision." This may enhance the ability to supervise others later on. In contrast, at the doctoral level, there is more room for planning, providing, and assessing. Doctoral students must defend the statement that "supervision is necessary for the development of clinical and professional skills."

The results showed that the master's students felt that the course allowed them to critique the supervision they receive. They reported being more aware of their own contributions as a supervisee. The doctoral students, on the other hand, felt as though the course allowed them to enhance their professional roles as supervisors.

Strategies

Some of the current strategies that are currently employed by researchers in the field of clinical supervision include metapragmatic awareness, reflective practice, and the use of personal narratives (Behrens et al., 2007; Geller & Foley, 2009; McCready & Raleigh, 2009): Each of these strategies contributes to the scientific underpinnings in this area of study and may be used to develop both supervisory competence as well as train clinical skills of a new clinician. It also should be noted that the use of research in this area is largely qualitative due to the individualized nature of supervision. However, there is a growth of cumulative evidence that is gained through these practices as well as knowledge of all available strategies which supports a scientific, evidence-based approach to supervision.

Research Tool #1: Conversational Analysis

The field of conversational analysis is one discipline which looks at and analyzes everyday conversations to undercover and describe how speakers achieve the structure and organization of conversation. One practical application of this research methodology is metapragmatic analysis, which is an evidence-based practice that enhances supervision through increased awareness of components of supervisory dialogues. Metapragmatic analysis (alternatively referred to as metapragmatic awareness throughout this chapter) examines speakers' attitudes about their own language behaviors (Behrens & Jablon, 2008). In fact, the mutual study of supervisory dialogues has revealed new knowledge about the process of clinical growth for both the supervisor and supervisee. Such perceptual data are useful for determining what each half of the dyad contributes in the conversation, given the opportunity to think about the use of the verbal behavior actually displayed, especially as the meaning of linguistic traits is contextual (Behrens & Jablon, 2008).

A pilot investigation led by Susan Behrens, Ph.D., (unpublished data) has contributed to the understanding of metapragmatic awareness as a tool in teacher training, with direct implications for speech-language clinicians and supervisors. In this study, portions of mid-semester and end-of semester supervisory conferences between entry-level students and supervisors were recorded. These data were subsequently transcribed and analyzed using the technique of conversational analysis. At the end of the semester, the students and supervisors listened to the recordings of their dialogues and asked to reflect on their thoughts and feelings regarding the interaction. They were asked to identify any specific factors that they felt played a role in the interaction, as well as their own conversational styles.

The results of this pilot study indicated that metapragmatic assessment was indeed a useful tool for improving self-awareness and the quality of the interaction between students and supervisors. This technique was extremely valuable in that the scrutiny of language skills used by the supervisor was found to be equally as important as the language skills used by the student clinicians in dealing with their clients. Results showed that there is a need to increase awareness of criteria and incongruence, especially across conversational partners. It is of interest that even trained supervisors are not necessarily aware of their own communicative styles.

The following are some excerpts as to what the metapragmatic assessment revealed. The following segment illustrates reflections by two different supervisors working with students who were either of the same age or older, where both were at different junctures in life.

Supervisor: When I'm the supervisor I think I try to make people my equal . . . the (student) is older than me and this is her second job and she's a mom and so she has a lot more life experience than I have. I just happen to have, you know, got my degree in Speech before she got her degree in Speech. And so in every other aspect it should completely be a role reversal, she should be my teacher in every other aspect of life probably, except this one.

Supervisor: I think that, you know, us being the same age actually has been beneficial because even though I took on the supervisory role to teach her things. I think that the peer interaction actually really did help because I wasn't talking to her as a young child and her not being way older than me, she wasn't looking at me as being a child or younger than her in that sense, even though I was in a supervisory position. So I think that that has definitely been beneficial in us working together.

I happened to be a participant in this particular study, thus the following example contains the metapragmatic assessment of myself and my student during a graduate externship.

Metapragmatic Assessment

Supervisor: It seems to me that the transcript reflects a good working relationship that I know this student and her work fairly well because we're confirming the things that she's done or been asked to do and she's agreeing that she's completed them and anticipated them actually, has done some in advance. There's a few less "um's" this time than in my other transcript. This particular student is um foreign accent, a foreign speaker, but she's able to follow like I would say like 98% of what I say speaking at a full rate of speech. I was aware sometimes of trying to repeat something or trying to re-clarify it to make sure that she understood it. I don't know if she used a lot of questioning if she did not under-stand. She was keeping on agreeing and we were pointing to a schedule so we were saying um mutual behaviors regarding that the clients are coming, which is their identification information. There probably was not really much controversy. She didn't really supply many questions in this transcript but I still felt that there was a good just general tone to it. I don't think we um needed to clarify too much back and forth on this, aware that I just said "um." I think that we were both equally partnering in this in terms of assertiveness or direction, we were both trying to reach a mutual goal and we really didn't have too much room for negotiating. But there was a good amount of give and take, my piece is not so much longer than her piece just visually looking at this and I feel satisfied.

From my current perspective, this was my first experience taping myself in supervision as opposed to taping students in training sessions. I feel that I learned a great deal from engaging in this process. It has greatly contributed to my understanding of how science can be applied to supervision and self-knowledge. It also has allowed me to reflect on my own clinical interaction style, which is something that had never been brought to my attention so pointedly, in all the years that I have been supervising.

The results of this unpublished research revealed by Behrens and colleagues (2007) revealed that many of the dyads expressed positive sentiments, and felt that the use of this approach was beneficial to them in terms of enhancing their self-awareness of clinical style. Furthermore, metapragmatic analysis appears to be a useful tool for developing supervisory skills of students and supervisors. It has the potential to prevent communication breakdowns and supports the establishment of rapport. The science of supervision is enhanced by knowledge that supervision takes different forms depending on characteristics of the supervisee, such as age, gender, language, culture, and other dynamics.

Additional Thoughts

This research is valuable in illustrating that the alignment of perceptions in an instructional dyad is critical to management of outcomes and expectations. The work of Hudson (2010) expanded the topic of supervision and mentorship, stating that although the student supervisor and CF (clinical fellow) mentor share many roles and responsibilities, there are key differences. Primarily, the mentor facilitates clinical independence through training techniques such as reflective practice. Factors such as interpersonal skills, cultural factors, and social power influence the mentorship models used. The application of learning models established by conversational analysis is a scientifically based methodology that can be applied to the considerations suggested by Behrens et al. (2007) above.

In addition, the guided use of self-assessment is very important in training young clinicians. The research contributed by McCarthy (2010) was very instructive in providing benchmarks for use in reflective practice. McCarthy's research focused on speech-language pathology graduate students and concluded that modifications to their practice were implemented when reflections were based on students' own clinical skills. Using performance indicators and written reflection conjointly enhanced clinical instruction. The research in supervision has contributed these results to be considered in the study and practice of clinical education.

Research Tool #2: Reflective Practice

Another strategy, developed from the work of Schon (1987), contributed to our understanding of thinking and learning. Schon's (1987) work on reflective practice has been used across disciplines and currently is being adapted for use in speech-pathology. Geller and Foley (2009) described the use of reflection as trained in mental health practice as a tool to enhance supervisory strategies. They put forth the notion that, traditionally, supervision in speech-language pathology has focused on discipline-specific training, with little emphasis on cognitive and affective domains. The advanced supervisor requires self-insight and is challenged to understand that his or her training of a less seasoned clinician is influenced by the quality of their relationship. Beyond the concrete aspects of the speech-language goals being trained, the supervisor must be attuned to psychodynamic factors at play during any communicative interaction. These underlying factors, such as concepts of transference of feelings between client and clinician, and countertransference of feelings, may be addressed in supervisory conferences to increase awareness of the dynamics between the triad of the client, clinician, and supervisor. In terms of science, this is a research construct, and it resonates with clinicians who have experienced personal dynamics between themselves and their client and supervisor that goes beyond the traditional learning objectives at hand.

Using exemplary scenarios, Geller and Foley (2009) demonstrate that there are several "ports of entry" to successful clinical communication. The supervisor has the ability to sensitize the clinician to working on external behaviors as well as internal motivations. The science of supervision is enhanced by this model by incorporating knowledge from interdisciplinary areas such as psychology, all of which contribute to a successful clinical experience.

Research Tool #3: Personal Narratives

McCready and Raleigh (2009) contribute another tool for scientific inquiry into what makes supervision successful. They place great emphasis on the notion that the supervisor must know him or herself and have a keen understanding and awareness of their personal philosophy as a teacher as well as a learner prior to teaching (supervising) another. According to McCready and Raleigh (2009), this may be accomplished by writing a directed self-analysis, or personal narrative, to gain a better understanding of ones' self. The authors suggest several key questions and concepts, which may be used as a guide, as follows:

1. What chapters, key events or turning points in my life have influenced the teacher/supervisor I am?

2. What is it about teaching/supervising that appeals to me?

3. What are the main ideas/underlying principles that characterize my teaching/supervising?

4. What educational and clinical goals do I set for my students or supervisees in accordance with my underlying principles?

5. What methods do I use to achieve these goals?

6. What are the sources from which I draw my teaching/supervising inspiration?

(Adapted from McCready & Raleigh, 2009.)

Important results can be obtained using techniques such as personal narrative writing, with significant effort, but the gains are multifold. Comments from students and supervisors who engage in written reflections regarding expectations and outcome strongly reflect personal and professional growth. Written reflections also provide a foundation by which others may model their career-long commitment to excellence.

In terms of my own practice, the use of a self-narrative is extremely important, and is one of the motives for this book. I have always been keenly aware not only of what I was teaching, but to whom I was teaching it. The use of personal inquiry is a step in scientific investigation as individual perspective colors the questions we have and how we seek the answers to those questions.

The science of supervision is enhanced by teaching these practices to new and seasoned clinicians and supervisors, as they have the potential to be beneficial for everyone. Engaging in the kind of work that professionals in this field do, it is important to always be cognizant of not only the client's present needs and state of mind, but also one's own. Self-reflection and evaluation is a life-long process, and one that is important to engage in if we are to move forward in life.

Supervision may include both written (personal narratives) and verbal reflections (metapragmatic assessment), as well as information sharing to increase awareness of interpersonal dynamics that are at play within the course of therapy. All of the techniques described above can be used either alone or in combination. They also may be applied meaningfully to enhance supervision across all levels of training, from beginning entry-level students to more experienced graduate-level students.

As described throughout this chapter, being a good supervisor calls on a great many more skills and competencies than simply textbook knowledge of the disorders and intervention strategies. Successful supervision and mentorship are both learned skills that require a great deal of self-reflection and awareness of a multitude of factors that are always at play in the supervisory dynamic. As such, in this chapter we outlined and discussed some of the competencies necessary to be a good supervisor. These include an understanding of interpersonal communication styles, cultural and linguistic factors, personal resilience, and sensitivity to "social power." We also looked at some current research strategies designed to increase the effectiveness of supervision, including narrative writing, metapragmatic awareness, and reflective practice. Part of being a good supervisor and clinician requires keeping up with the current thinking in the field. As such, it is very important that supervisors keep themselves abreast of current trends so as to strive for continuous personal and professional growth and development.

What's Next?

In the next chapter we examine another critical issue that currently is taking center stage in our field—evidence-based practice.

Reflective Assignment

Use the questions below to guide you in your thinking and writing of a personal narrative/supervision philosophy.

1. What chapters, key events, or turning points in my life have influenced the mentor/supervisor that I am today?

2. What is it about teaching/supervising that appeals to me?

3. What are the main ideas/underlying principles that characterize my mentoring/supervising?

4. What educational and clinical goals do I set for my students or supervisees in accordance with my underlying principles?

5. What methods do I use to achieve these goals?

6. What are the sources from which I draw my teaching/supervising inspiration?

(Adapted from McCready & Raleigh, 2009.)

CHAPTER 7

Evidence-Based Practice: Interplay Between Research and Practice

Research is to see what everybody else has seen, and to think what nobody else has thought.

William Osler

The Need for Evidence-Based Practice

All of the information contained in the previous chapters contributes to the establishment and upholding of evidence-based practice (EBP) within our field. According to ASHA (2005), evidence-based practice is the integration of: (a) clinical expertise, (b) best current evidence, and (c) client/patient perspectives to provide high-quality services reflecting the interests, values, needs, and choices of the individuals we serve. According to Sackett et al. (1996), EBP is the integration of best research evidence with clinical expertise and client values.

There has been an increased emphasis on, and call for, evidence-based practice in our field over the course of the past several years. Incorporating evidence-based practice into our treatment is another way of ejecting the scientific principles of data analysis and outcome measures into our field, in an effort to establish a base for the efficacy of treatment techniques and strategies.

It is our professional responsibility to make sure that we apply these principles to both clinical care and supervision. We are encouraged to do so by evaluating the efficacy, effectiveness, and efficiency of clinical protocols for treatment; monitoring and incorporating new and high-quality evidence into our practice; and carefully evaluating all diagnostic and treatment procedures (ASHA, 2005).

Why is evidence-based practice continuously necessary? There is a need in all professional practice areas that address human behavior to continuously integrate new information. Furthermore, new needs continue to arise in all areas of clinical practice that require theoretical principles as the foundation for establishing sound practice (in other words, to show that theory can be successfully applied to practice). As such, investigation of available research helps practitioners to understand the literature in a deeper fashion. Thus, in an effort to incorporate these principles into practice with clients, an actively engaged practitioner must serve as an advocate for advancing knowledge both on one's own part and that of the professionals (both novice and experienced) under his or her charge. Recently, a growing database of research supporting evidence-based practice is present in the speech-pathology literature.

Applying Evidence-Based Practice to Supervision Research

The science of supervision is enhanced through the application of evidence-based strategies that are used in researching clinical questions. The use of prior clinical examples, guided self-reflection, careful consideration of language style, and modification of cultural aspects are all examples of embedding evidence-based practice into supervision. The science of successful supervision and mentorship is furthered by an evidence-based approach including data collected in the field and cumulative knowledge, which is subject to specific variations driven by the particular setting, practitioners' experience, and clients' preference.

This is in keeping with evidence-based research that seeks to analyze appropriate data and then make modifications based on individual factors which are taken into account. The research done by many ASHA members individually as well as in the Special Interest Division on Administration and Supervision is reported in this book, alongside the clinical experience of the present author.

Kelly, Kingma, and Robinson (2010), reported on a method to assist in the evaluation of clinical and research evidence that can be adapted to supervision literature. Their methodology involved the development of the research question, citation, design/method, participants, experimental group, controls, results, analysis of strengths and weaknesses, and level of evidence in a format for clinicians to use in their individual settings. The structured reading of literature focuses the supervisory education of clinicians to evaluate evidence in this practice area.

The steps to practicing evidence based self-monitoring of supervision and mentorship can be adapted using the principles of research methodology. The background of this situation lies in the ability of students and clinicians, as well as potential supervisors and mentors, to engage deeply in critical thinking and problem-based learning. Critical thinking and challenging evaluative assumptions are important in clinical decision-making. These skills are also integral to the management of a large caseload and the needs of families, subordinates, peers, and other professionals throughout a meaningful career.

One recent article, "Problem-Based Learning, Critical Thinking and Concept Mapping in Speech-Language Pathology Education: A Review," by Mok, Whitehill, and Dodd (2008) emphasizes the importance of graduate schools engaging students in problem-based learning, which will lead to better integration between theory and practice—the underlying issue in seeking the evidence-based approach.

It is important for clinical supervisors to utilize several different sources of research compilations in order to provide relevant meta-analyses regarding case areas under study. There currently are several such information databases, including the Cochrane Library, the Agency for Healthcare Research and Quality (http://www.gu ideline.gov), the National Institute on Deafness and Other Communication Disorders, and the Academy of Neurological Communication Disorders and Sciences. The American Speech-Language Hearing

Association has also compiled a comprehensive list of both guidelines and systematic reviews in evidence-based practice, which have been divided into different areas (ASHA/N-CEP Evidence-Based Systematic Reviews, 2010c).

Types of Evidence

There are different types of evidence that a clinician or supervisor may encounter. These include the evidence gained from review of relevant literature, from clinical practice, and from preferences expressed by clients or by colleagues. However, it is important to note that clinical judgment alone is not considered enough data to support the efficacy of using a specific approach or methodology, even for the most experienced clinicians.

A clinician also should possess sufficient training to analyze the material they read. Students at the graduate level generally are required to take a research methods course in order to complete educational requirements. However, the challenges of a fulltime professional career may render it impossible for clinicians to utilize a hypothesis-testing approach to the cases they treat. Thus, many SLP's develop greater skills in application of theory rather than in testing the scientific method. Yet, all of our work should be based on methods that have likelihood to succeed based on the probability outcomes of large randomized trials. And although there currently is great emphasis being placed on evidence-based practice, this is not yet accomplished in many of the helping professions.

In terms of the value of scientific research, it is critical that clinicians at all levels of practice look at sound data to support clinical decisions. Well-controlled scientific studies help us to make improved critical opinions regarding the phenomena we see in our clients and ourselves. In its purest sense, empirical research implies that the outcome obtained is due to no exogenous variable other than the procedure being tested, as all other factors were "controlled." Speech-language pathology and clinical supervision is grounded in sound underlying findings. Clinical efficacy research is also an undertaking by ASHA in their large National Outcomes

Measurement Surveys (NOMS) programs. Information gained by clinical experience must be met with advances in theoretical knowledge to maintain professional relevance.

Usefulness of Evidence-Based Practice

The usefulness of research driven approaches to practice and supervision are clear. In any situation that collects public monies or compensation from a third party, there is a need for accountability. This also extends to private pay situations whereby clinicians' practice depends on efficiency of outcome. We should be seeking evidence to support our clinical decisions from the first encounter with a client and/or junior clinician. Based on evidence, a skilled clinician should ideally have some idea of what strategies she or he is most likely to employ with a given disorder (or several treatment options, to see which may work best), and what to expect at three month intervals of evaluation. The same holds true for clinical supervision, although the data are not as readily available.

Systematized controlled studies of interpersonal communication contacts can start with data-driven observations about the individuals in the supervisory dyad, the case in question, and the purposes of the supervision. Expectations and outcomes should be planned with measures such as attitude surveys and questionnaires that can be self-developed at the outset. The reliability and validity of these tools would require ongoing assessment and may be able to be adapted for local norms measurement after a period of careful study.

Levels of Evidence

On the one hand, medicine is accumulating many meta-analyses of clinical trials and other types of studies under Cochrane's International Library database by which physicians and other interested parties can research "what works" and "what doesn't." A recent search reveals, incidentally, that there are a handful of reviews of speech therapy with some of the major diagnostic groups; with the majority finding being that it is inconclusive whether or not speech intervention is effective.

To move forward in our understanding of both specific client driven methodologies as well as what may work in supervision, it is important to have an understanding of the "strength of evidence" standard in this expert opinion. Robey (2004) describes the examples of evidence level according to the source of the evidence, which is then assigned a classification.

The highest level of evidence "1A" is the meta-analysis of multiple well-designed controlled studies. The next level of evidence "1" consists of well-designed randomized controlled trials. Well-designed nonrandomized controlled trials constitute level "2." Level "3" evidence consists of observational studies using control variables, and level "4" evidence is the observational studies without controls. The Health Care research guidelines provide an additional category, "Good Practice Points," in which there is lack of finite evidence but good consensus among clinical practitioners evaluating the study in question.

Research Design

In supervision research, the single-subject research design may be most appropriate as compared to group research design. The aim of a single-subject design is to analyze the performance of an individual subject in each condition tested. There are two stages of single-subject designs. The first is the baseline of initial behavioral observation (A), followed by the treatment segment in which the independent variable is being manipulated (B). This is traditionally referred to as an "A-B" design.

A variation of this design is the "ABA" design in which the baseline is reexamined after the "treatment" interval to determine if there is a return to baseline levels of function once treatment is completed or removed. Finally, there is the "ABAB" design which consists of a baseline and treatment followed by a second baseline and treatment. If the treatment is effective, there should be a return in the second baseline to pretreatment conditions and then a change in function after treatment is re-initiated. Single-subject designs can be helpful in systematically tracking changes in individual behavior over time and to examine effects of applying a particular treatment paradigm.

There can be distinct advantages for speech-language pathology supervisors to employ single-subject design methodologies when establishing and evaluating supervisory practices and paradigms as there likely are only a small number of subjects. This avoids subject matching issues, which may not be appropriate or practical in clinical supervision. This methodology is flexible and meaningful if interpreted within the context of single-subject design and case study research, which has precedence in our field. It is of significant importance to emphasize that the results can in no way be generalized as those obtained in large group designs and as such, we must approach the level 3 of evidence.

Integrating Principles of Evidence-Based Practice Across Training Levels

Christine Dollaghan (2007) has made a very important contribution to speech-language pathology evidence-gathering as it pertains to practice and the profession at-large. In an effort to bring this information to supervision and mentorship, the following is a an entry observation on how to apply some of the principles discussed above into a scientific approach to supervision, which goes beyond the case presentation and feedback discussion paradigm of the earlier years of the profession; and undoubtedly in use today in many meaningful contexts.

Throughout our experiences early on in our training, we know that there is 100% supervision required in the initial undergraduate clinic experience, and that students may only interact with a case after 25 hours of observation. However, different programs handle the initial practicum in varying ways. In one university program, which participated in a feedback survey for this chapter, the Director of the program indicates that the faculty is attempting to move toward the direction of evidence-based practice instruction. They accomplish this in several ways. In one course, students are asked to conduct an independent literature search and create an annotated bibliography of research supporting therapeutic approaches for specific disorders. The students also may be required to provide a research article describing the treatment approach for any clients they are assigned in the clinic.

At the undergraduate level, the students are not asked to assess the research for level of evidence. However, the process of, and acclimation to, gathering of research for clinical rationales and efficacy data is the important first step in all treatment design. Unfortunately, this level of commitment to research typically is not carried over when students are sent out to do their externships in outside facilities. Thus, this level of information is lost on many students when they are no longer required to conduct such thorough research for coursework and hence, the meaningfulness of the use of evidence may not be clear to novice clinicians who were not trained in this fashion.

Clinical Walk-Through: Graduate Student and Clinical Supervisor

The case scenario below illustrates how evidence-based practice can be incorporated into a dialogue with an entry-level clinician during a supervisory conference. This student has been given her first caseload, which includes 2 young clients, ages 3 and 5, both of whom present with severe articulation issues.

> Student: Should I bring materials or follow the previous clinicians' plans to follow up? Will I be doing the session alone or will you help me?

> Supervisor: Have you ever worked with these types of clients before? Have you had any classes that discussed these issues?

> Student: I've observed a few, but have never independently led a session.

> Supervisor: I have a really good article. Let's read it together for next week before you see the clients. Using what you've

read, why don't you try to come up with 1 or 2 activities and we can discuss them next time we meet.

This simple scenario calls on introducing the entry level students with using available literature as a starting point in intervention. The supervisor would encourage the student clinician to observe how the client may fit in with the profile described and where there may be individual differences. In addition, the supervisor would encourage a careful history and parent interview to determine case specifics and client preferences. Later stage supervision might include comparing another article regarding the depth of research and applicability between the two research articles to begin to teach comparison of levels of evidence.

Another suggestion to remedy this problem is to use a group case study, which can act as an initial starting point. A simple design might look like Table 7-1.

Table 7–1. EBP—Group Case Study Project

Relevant Background and Analysis		
Above Average	**Average**	**Below Average**
Offers own analysis using levels of evidence approach, reaching conclusion	Mostly incomplete analysis	Poor choice of references, no analysis possible
Disorder and Theoretical Inquiry		
Above Average	**Average**	**Below Average**
Gives strong clinical examples and relevant support	Repetitive information from case history; little independent assessment	Selects irrelevant behaviors to report, ineffective examples
ASSESSMENT—Points _____ / 100 Grade _____		

Source: Adapted from Queen's University Belfast (2010). *Note:* This particular document contains many useful case study applications and the interested reader is referred to the original document.

Group learning may help facilitate the growth of students and supervisors. A place to begin could be team building within the student mentees and between the mentees and supervisor. The benefit of working with a team approach is that it can facilitate the application of knowledge. It also can increase implicit learning that otherwise may not be attainable in traditional curriculum. Morrison, Lincoln and Reed (2009) contrasted American students to Australian students. They found that Australians rated themselves higher on knowledge about teamwork. In contrast, Americans had higher ratings on attitudes toward teams, but all students perceived they had the skills to work on teams. Using this information as a fact finding base, it is possible to begin an evidence-gathering project among the students regarding relevant topics and a supervisory self-study as a starting point of systematic self-evaluation. An example follows:

CHART/EXERCISE

In terms of individual practice, the supervisor-mentor must

1	Formulate a clear question relative to his/her practice.
2	Identify research that answers question or relevant aspects.
3	Critically evaluate the pertinent literature.
4	Apply the evidence gained to clinical practice.
5	Re-evaluate application of evidence at periodic intervals.

Borrowing from other areas, a simplified approach to understanding research articles can be applied for the novice supervisor-mentor seeking to expand their knowledge of relevant literature to improve their own practice. This includes:

1. Define the area of patient diagnosis or case management issue to be examined

2. Apply an intervention based on available research

3. Compare results using standards of pretest–intervention–posttest

4. Determine outcome of efficacy

(Adapted from Zakowski, Seibert, & VanEyck, 2004)

In appraising relevant research, several questions should be examined. They include whether the subject group was carefully controlled; was the result related directly and solely to the intervention in question; what other factors might explain the results?

As a practice exercise, readers may want to write their own clinical case study of a supervision scenario using the outline below:

EBP—Supervision Practice Case Study

Supervisor:

Clinician:

Dilemma:

Factors:

Known information:

What needs to be known:

Sources of information:

Desired outcomes:

Relevant research:

Practice With Levels of Evidence

Practice writing these elements using real or hypothetical situations and developing several outcomes and rank order, and discuss feasibility. This can be used in supervisory meetings or in instructional workshops. By not supplying all of the information and instead having clinicians develop their own scenarios, this enables practitioners to improve their independent clinical decision-making. They become more independent at accumulating and defending opinions based on the literature.

Doing these types of training exercises can be beneficial for both beginning clinicians and professionals who have been in the field for many years. By better preparing senior personnel for supervision, we are initiating a trickle-down effect from the top-down enhancing the entire service delivery system. Saras and Post (2004) point out that SLP supervision styles may mirror those of general education supervisors. As a profession, we must distinguish between the behaviors a supervisor must possess and those they are expected to display, so that we offer exemplary practice and make more standard responses to critical teaching scenarios.

The need for enhanced personnel preparation in speech-language pathology has been incrementally affected by the increased complexities of caseloads, roles, and responsibilities of speech-language pathologists. We no longer can train generalists. The critical shortage of qualified speech-language pathologists and the faculty to train them, has implications for curricula, clinical training, and research (Whitmire & Eger, 2003; 2004).

In conclusion, if a clinician-supervisor chose to begin his or her review of this area using a comparative literature approach, considerable research sophistication is necessary. Although this topic may go beyond the scope of this book, the reader is encouraged to refer to the work of Robey and Dalebout (1998). The authors provide a "tutorial" on how meta-analysis can best design reviews of studies. Numerical comparisons of effect size can be calculated meaningfully if review articles themselves are well-constructed and the design of the meta-analysis follows suit. Threats to interpretation of the outcome can follow from flaws in the design of the variable and measurements, as well as failure to account for other factors effecting outcomes, just as in individual designs.

In this chapter we looked at the principles of evidence-based practice and how they can be applied to supervision research. Evidence-based practice is a newer area in speech-language pathology and is still being applied to disorders. The application of evidence-based practice to supervision is new ground in speech-language pathology. Yet, it is the essence of care in that treatment outcome may depend on effective supervision, and therefore warrants as much or greater attention as that which we apply to each area of clinical practice.

We outlined and discussed the different levels of evidence that a supervisor may use, and how to incorporate these into training students of different levels using clinical scenarios and case study examples. It would require a consensus among present and future practitioners to appreciate the scientific aspects that have been studied in supervision to date.

What's Next?

In the following chapter, we take a closer look at mentorship and some of the issues and challenges that we face as mentors.

CHAPTER 8

Insights Into Mentorship and Supervision

Mentoring is a brain to pick, an ear to listen, and a push in the right direction.

John Crosby

What Is Mentorship?

Clark and Johnson (2000), who describe mentorship in psychology programs, state that mentors provide two primary functions: those fulfilling career goals and those fulfilling psychosocial goals. In general, there are five distinct characteristics of mentoring relationships according to the authors. A mentoring relationship is a helping relationship designed to achieve both long- and short-term goals. Mentoring is aimed at achieving professional and psychological growth. It is a reciprocal relationship which is both professional and personal. The mentor is always the person who is in the greater professional sphere of influence and experience.

Furthermore, it is conceivable that: (1) mentors are not in the same primary field as the mentee and (2) mentorship information may cross over to other professional disciplines. This article's contribution to empirical information is considered highly relevant to this discussion. Although Clark and Johnson (2000) suggest that there is scant research information on this topic, it is clear that a mentor plays a more significant role than a supervisor. However, this is not meant to undermine the role of either party, as both contribute greatly to a student's growth and development. A supervisor seeks to encourage and enhance the development of a practitioner within the requirements of their position in an organization. On the other hand, a mentor seeks to develop the mentee in a much broader life and professional construct, regardless of the particular workplace setting.

Although the concept of close mentorship is somewhat outmoded by modern exigencies, the need for personal and professional nurturance continues. Some modern exigencies include economic demands to produce, technologic competitiveness, as well as time and labor constraints. In speech-language pathology, we lag behind related disciplines such as psychology in terms of studying this topic as a means of adding to our knowledge base of evidence-based practice. However, as described in subsequent chapters, there currently is more research being conducted. It is important to note that even within psychology, a lead discipline examining this area, there is a need for greater evidence about the requirements of a mentor and mentoring relationships. Factors such as gender, race, and ethnic matching are criteria that may be relevant to examine in terms of predicting success in setting up mentoring programs.

Research indicates that some of the primary personal characteristics ascribed to effective mentors have included supportiveness, intelligence, knowledge, ethics, caring, humor, and encouraging manner. These are consistent with informal data obtained by the author from students in speech-language pathology. As mentorship is not required in most of the practice professions, not all students or professionals have mentors. Consequently, some may have had multiple mentors. In this sense, the definition of what constitutes a mentor and a mentoring relationship may be obscured by the operational definitions used within various programs of study. Of those who are not mentored or not mentored well, it leads to questions about characteristics of mentorship.

In some cases, there may be a relationship between the personal security of an individual and their ability to seek and engage in an open mentoring relationship. It may be possible that those who need it most may not pursue mentoring for a host of factors related to individual background and culture. In general, those who are mentored tend to express greater outcomes of success and satisfaction than those who are not. According to Clark and Johnson's

(2000) work, there is a significant degree of difference between those who receive mentoring and those who do not. They pose that a lack of mentorship, and/or poor mentoring may lead to early exit from programs before achieving completion. It is clear by their report that good mentorship may lead to enhancements in professional identity, confidence, and opportunities.

Mentorship Versus Supervision

According to most informants, there are major differences between supervision and mentorship. Clinical supervision in speech-language pathology follows a standard of sequential training. This training is guided by curriculum, clinical instruction, and close supervision through the period when the clinician obtains certification and independent licensure. In many departments, there also continues to be a supervisory function that becomes more administrative as clinicians develop professional experience. Many departments choose to develop an ongoing collaboration with information sharing, case progress, and continuing education activities. Licensed professionals are legally and ethically responsible for their own activities. Professionals benefit from continued exposure to education and opportunities to supervise clinical interns and externs.

A typical prototype of supervision encompasses ASHA standards as well as the site-specific requirements. As an example, the Burlington-Edison School District (2010) developed a comprehensive rubric in order to enhance professional practice in domains such as preparation and planning (Table 8-1). The goal of the rubric is clearly designed to enhance professional practice in their site-specific special education setting. However, it clearly can be adapted for use in other settings as well as by individuals seeking to improve professional competence in the form of self-supervision and mentorship. This demonstrates that training and education can continue very meaningfully even after formal training is completed.

Table 8–1. Rubrics for Enhancing Professional Practice: Speech/Language Pathologist

DOMAINS: #1 PLANNING AND PREPARATION

ELEMENT	UNSATISFACTORY	BASIC	PROFICIENT	DISTINGUISHED
1a: Demonstrating Knowledge of Content and Pedagogy [Speech and Language Development and Procedures for Correction]	Therapist displays little understanding of prerequisite knowledge of content and pedagogic issues, and makes content errors or does not correct students' errors.	Therapist displays content knowledge and awareness of prerequisite learning and pedagogic knowledge, but knowledge is incomplete and not connected with other parts of the discipline.	Therapist displays knowledge, planning reflects understanding of relationships and pedagogic practices reflect current research on best practices.	Therapist displays content knowledge, actively builds on knowledge of prerequisite relationships, displays continuing search for best practice, and anticipates students' difficulties.
1b: Demonstrating Knowledge of Students on Caseload	Therapist displays minimal knowledge of speech and language developmental characteristics of age group and is unfamiliar with learning approaches, student's skills and knowledge, cultural heritage, and interests.	Therapist has knowledge of speech and language developmental characteristics and general understanding of learning approaches while recognizing value of knowing students' skills, interests, and cultural heritage.	Therapist displays thorough understanding of speech and language developmental characteristics and different approaches to learning, and knowledge of students' skills, interests, and cultural heritage.	Therapist displays knowledge of students' speech and language developmental characteristics, skills, knowledge, interests, and cultural heritage and varies approaches in instructional planning appropriate to individual students.

106

ELEMENT	UNSATISFACTORY	BASIC	PROFICIENT	DISTINGUISHED
1c: Selecting Instructional Goals	Goals are not clear, do not reflect current evaluation and IEP, are not suitable for the instructional setting, reflect only one type of learning, represent low expectations for the students, and do not permit viable methods of assessment and do not reflect alignment with EALRs or GLEs.	Goals are moderately valuable, clear, and consistent with current IEP and evaluation, reflecting several types of learning, most are suitable for most students, sometimes reflect alignment with EALRs and GLEs, but some do not permit viable methods of assessment.	Goals are clear, with valuable expectations, clearly reflect current evaluation and IEP, reflect several types of learning opportunities and are suitable for most students, usually reflect alignment with EALRs and GLEs, and most permit viable methods of assessment.	Goals are valuable, establish high expectations, clearly reflect current evaluation and IEP, are clearly articulated, reflect student initiative, account for different learning needs, reflect alignment with EALRs and GLEs, and permit viable methods of assessment.
1d: Designing Coherent Instruction, Therapy Session, and Structure	Learning activities are not suitable for students or IEP goals. They do not follow an organized progression and do not reflect recent professional practice.	Only some of the learning activities are suitable to students or IEP goals. Progression of activities is uneven, and only some activities reflect recent professional practice.	Most of the learning activities are suitable to students and IEP goals. Progression of activities is fairly even, and most activities reflect recent professional practice.	Learning activities are highly relevant to students and IEP goals. They progress coherently, producing a unified whole and reflecting recent professional research and practice.

continues

Table 8–1. *continued*

DOMAINS: #2 EVALUATION/ASSESSMENT

ELEMENT	UNSATISFACTORY	BASIC	PROFICIENT	DISTINGUISHED
2a: Collection of Information	Usually requires supervisory guidance to accurately select case history or other interview formats with consideration for all relevant factors. SLP collects case history information that is incomplete or lacking in relevance. SLP is unable to integrate data to identify etiologic and/or contributing factors.	Sometimes requires supervisory guidance to accurately select case history or other interview formats with consideration for all relevant factors. SLP may collect case history information that is incomplete or lacking in relevance. SLP may be unable to integrate data to identify etiologic and/ or contributing factors.	In most situations, SLP independently and accurately selects case history or other interview formats with consideration for all relevant factors. SLP collects and probes student/family for additional information, obtains information from other sources, and integrates data to identify etiologic and/or contributing factors.	Independently and accurately selects case history or other interview formats with consideration for all relevant factors. SLP efficiently collects pertinent information from the student/ family spontaneously probes for additional relevant information, obtains information from other sources, and integrates data in order to identify etiologic and/or contributing factors to develop comprehensive student profile.

ELEMENT	UNSATISFACTORY	BASIC	PROFICIENT	DISTINGUISHED
2b: Selection of Evaluation/ Assessment Materials	Requires supervisory guidance to select evaluation/ assessment procedures that are appropriate and complete. SLP requires assistance with consideration of relevant factors. Assessment/ evaluation materials do not answer question of concern. SLP may administer and/or score tests inaccurately or incompletely.	Usually requires some supervisory guidance to select evaluation/ assessment procedures that are appropriate and complete. SLP requires assistance with consideration of relevant factors. SLP may administer and/or score tests inaccurately or incompletely.	SLP independently selects an adequate evaluation/ assessment battery (i.e., basic procedures needed to define problem adequately) with consideration for most relevant factors. SLP administers the battery and consistently scores tests accurately.	Independently selects a comprehensive evaluation/ assessment battery with consideration for all relevant factors. SLP efficiently and accurately administers the battery and consistently scores tests accurately.

continues

Table 8–1. *continued*

ELEMENT	UNSATISFACTORY	BASIC	PROFICIENT	DISTINGUISHED
2c: Adaptation of Evaluation	Usually requires supervisory guidance to recognize the need for adaptations/ modifications. SLP consistently requires assistance in adapting procedures to accommodate individual and/or unique student needs, including communication variations such as cultural and linguistic diversity, limited English proficiency, etc.	Sometimes requires supervisory guidance to recognize the need for and/or adapt procedures to accommodate individual and/or unique student needs, including communication variations such as cultural and linguistic diversity, limited English proficiency, etc.	In most situations, SLP independently and accurately recognizes when testing procedures need to be adapted to accommodate needs unique to specific students and implements appropriate modifications. May need assistance in accessing available resources, including communication variations such as cultural and linguistic diversity, limited English proficiency, etc.	Independently and accurately recognizes when testing procedures need to be adapted to accommodate needs unique to specific students. SLP effectively implements appropriate adaptations and makes maximum use of all available resources to provide for unusual circumstances, including communication variations such as cultural and linguistic diversity, limited English proficiency, etc.

110

ELEMENT	UNSATISFACTORY	BASIC	PROFICIENT	DISTINGUISHED
2d: Interprets and Integrates Test Results	Usually requires supervisory guidance to interpret diagnostic data and/or behavioral observations accurately. SLP consistently requires supervisory assistance in defining student's level of communicative functioning. Diagnostic impressions and/or recommendations are either inappropriate, inconsistent with evaluation results, or absent.	Sometimes requires supervisory guidance to interpret diagnostic data and/or behavioral observations accurately in order to define the student's communicative functioning. Diagnostic impressions and/or recommendations may be inappropriate, inconsistent with evaluation results, or absent.	In most situations, SLP independently and accurately interprets and integrates test results and behavioral observations to define the student's communicative functioning. SLP develops diagnostic impressions and makes basic recommendations that are consistent with evaluation results and that are adequate for case.	Consistently, independently, and accurately interprets and integrates test results and behavioral observations to define the student's communicative functioning, which includes relating etiologic factors to observed behaviors and test results. SLP consistently develops diagnostic impressions and makes comprehensive recommendations leading to appropriate case management.

continues

Table 8–1. *continued*

DOMAINS: #3 TREATMENT/INTERVENTION

ELEMENT	UNSATISFACTORY	BASIC	PROFICIENT	DISTINGUISHED
3a: Develops and Implements Treatment Plans	Usually requires supervisory guidance to accurately develop a treatment plan appropriate for the student. The treatment plan may include adequate long-term goals, but objectives do not reflect logical sequencing of learned steps. SLP does not identify appropriate service delivery options, and even with guidance, does not demonstrate ability to effectively implement treatment plans.	Sometimes requires supervisory guidance to accurately develop a treatment plan appropriate for the student. The treatment plan may include adequate long-term goals, but objectives may not reflect logical sequencing of learned steps. SLP may not identify appropriate service delivery options, and requires supervision to effectively implement treatment plans.	In most situations, SLP independently and accurately establishes treatment plans appropriate for the student. The treatment plan includes long-term goals and short-term objectives, which usually reflect a logical sequencing of learning steps. SLP generally explores alternative service delivery options, but may need help in selecting the most appropriate options. SLP can effectively implement planned procedures.	Independently and accurately establishes a treatment plan appropriate for the student. SLP consistently develops specific and reasonable treatment plans that include long-term goals and short-term objectives which reflect appropriate learning sequence; explores all alternative service delivery options, identifies the most appropriate settings for service, and effectively implements plans.

112

ELEMENT	UNSATISFACTORY	BASIC	PROFICIENT	DISTINGUISHED
3b: Develops and Implements Intervention Strategies	Usually requires supervisory guidance to select/develop and implement intervention strategies relevant to the disorder and needs of the student.	Sometimes requires supervisory guidance to select/develop and implement intervention strategies relevant to the disorder and/or needs of the student.	In most situations, SLP independently selects/develops and implements intervention strategies relevant to the communication disorder and the unique characteristics of the student.	Independently selects/develops and implements comprehensive intervention strategies that take into consideration all unique characteristics and communication needs of the student.
3c: Selection and Use of Procedures	Usually requires supervisory guidance to recognize the need for adaptation of intervention procedures, strategies, materials, and/or instrumentation to accommodate needs unique to specific students.	Requires some supervisory guidance to recognize the need for adaptation of intervention procedures, strategies, materials, and/or instrumentation to accommodate needs unique to specific students.	Recognizes when intervention procedures, strategies, materials, and/or instrumentation need to be adapted to accommodate needs unique to specific students.	Independently and consistently adapts intervention procedures, strategies, materials, and instrumentation to accommodate needs unique to specific students.

continues

Table 8–1. *continued*

ELEMENT	UNSATISFACTORY	BASIC	PROFICIENT	DISTINGUISHED
3c: Selection and Use of Procedures *continued*	SLP demonstrates difficulty implementing identified adaptations and does not seek supervisory guidance when needed.	SLP may have difficulty implementing identified adaptations and may not consistently seek supervisory guidance when needed.	May use available resources for unusual circumstances. May need assistance in making appropriate adaptations.	Makes maximum use of all available resources to provide for unusual circumstances. SLP effectively implements appropriate adaptations.
3d: Selection and Use of Materials	Usually requires supervisory guidance to select materials and/or instrumentation that are appropriate to the treatment objectives, student, and/or the activity. SLP requires supervision to use materials and/or instrumentation effectively.	Requires some supervisory guidance to select materials and/or instrumentation that are appropriate to the treatment objectives, student, and/or the activity. Once selected, SLP may not use materials and/or instrumentation effectively.	In most cases, SLP independently selects/develops materials and instrumentation that are relevant to the communication disorder and uses materials and/or instrumentation effectively.	Independently and consistently selects/ develops materials and instrumentation with basis for clear rationale, and uses these materials and instrumentation creatively and effectively to enhance the treatment process.

ELEMENT	UNSATISFACTORY	BASIC	PROFICIENT	DISTINGUISHED
3e: Utilizes Therapy Time Effectively	Usually requires supervisory guidance to establish efficient use of direct therapy time. SLP requires assistance in preparation and adaptation of materials and utilization of therapy behavioral supports. Data collection procedures are not relevant to objectives and scheduling of therapy sessions may be ineffective for student needs. Objective(s) are not evident for therapy session(s).	Sometimes requires supervisory guidance to generate efficient use of direct therapy time. SLP may need assistance in preparation and adaptation of materials, use of therapy behavioral supports, organization of relevant data collection procedures, and scheduling of therapy sessions. Objective(s) may be clearly evident for each therapy session.	In most cases, SLP independently demonstrates efficient use of direct therapy time through preparation and adaptation of appropriate materials, use of appropriate behavioral supports, organization of relevant data collection procedures, and scheduling of therapy sessions. SLP usually demonstrates clearly evident objective(s) for each therapy session.	Independently and consistently demonstrates efficient use of direct therapy time through preparation and adaptation of appropriate materials, use of appropriate behavioral supports, organization of relevant data collection procedures, and scheduling of therapy sessions. SLP demonstrates clearly evident objective(s) for each therapy session.

continues

115

Table 8–1. *continued*

ELEMENT	UNSATISFACTORY	BASIC	PROFICIENT	DISTINGUISHED
3f: Establishes Rapport	Interactions with students are negative or inappropriate. Standards of conduct are not evident; students do not appear engaged; and student behavior is not monitored.	Interactions with students are generally appropriate. Standards of conduct appear to have been established; students are not consistently engaged; and student behavior is monitored infrequently.	Interactions with students are friendly, positive, and respectful. Standards of conduct are consistently established; students are usually engaged; and student behavior is frequently monitored.	Interactions with students are friendly, positive, respectful, and dynamic. Standards of conduct are clearly and consistently established; students are actively engaged; and student behavior is consistently monitored.

DOMAINS: #4 COORDINATING/COLLABORATING FUNCTIONS

ELEMENT	UNSATISFACTORY	BASIC	PROFICIENT	DISTINGUISHED
4a: Collaborates with Other Professionals	SLP usually requires supervisory guidance to effectively identify the need to consult or collaborate with other professionals regarding case management activities. SLP does not make decisions based on shared information, contribute and/or focus on mutual problem-solving activities.	SLP sometimes requires supervisory guidance to effectively identify the need to consult or collaborate with other professionals regarding case management activities. SLP does not make decisions based on shared information, contribute and/or focus on mutual problem-solving activities.	In most situations, SLP appropriately identifies the need to consult or collaborate with other professionals regarding case management activities. SLP listens carefully to input from others, makes appropriate decisions based on shared information, and usually participates in activities and contributes information that promotes mutual problem-solving.	SLP independently and consistently identifies the need to consult or collaborate with other professionals regarding case management activities. SLP consistently listens carefully to input from others, makes appropriate decisions based on shared information, initiates activities, and contributes information that promotes mutual problem-solving.

continues

Table 8–1. *continued*

ELEMENT	UNSATISFACTORY	BASIC	PROFICIENT	DISTINGUISHED
4b: Works Cooperatively	SLP is not available to staff for questions and/or assistance. Does not consult with others nor provide knowledge or understanding of material.	SLP is rarely available to staff for questions and/or assistance. May consult with others or provide knowledge or understanding of material.	SLP is available to staff and welcomes questions. Discusses professional subjects with staff from basic knowledge and collaborates with others when addressing student needs.	SLP often engages and is engaged with the staff in discussion about topics of concern to the staff. Spends as much time listening as speaking. Helps others to understand knowledge.
4c: Identifies and Refers Students for Services	SLP usually requires supervisory guidance to identify the need for student referrals and/or to make appropriate referrals.	SLP requires some supervisory guidance to identify the need for student referrals and/or to make appropriate referrals and seeks assistance in locating specific resources when appropriate.	SLP usually identifies the need for and makes student referrals, and seeks assistance in locating specific resources when appropriate.	SLP consistently identifies the need for and makes appropriate student referrals, and locates specific resources when appropriate.

DOMAINS: #5 COMMUNICATION SKILLS

ELEMENT	UNSATISFACTORY	BASIC	PROFICIENT	DISTINGUISHED
5a: Communicates Effectively	SLP does not present information accurately, logically, and concisely. Oral communication is not appropriate for the needs of the audience. SLP uses terminology and phrasing inconsistent with the semantic competence of the audience and includes information that is inaccurate and/or incomplete.	SLP intermittently presents information accurately, logically, and concisely. Oral communication is rarely appropriate and terminology and phrasing are often inconsistent with the semantic competency of the audience. SLP usually includes information that is accurate and/or complete.	SLP usually presents information accurately, clearly, logically, and concisely. Oral communication is appropriate in most situations, using terminology and phrasing consistent with the semantic competency of the audience. SLP includes information that is accurate and/or complete.	SLP independently presents information accurately, clearly, logically, and concisely. Oral communication is always appropriate for the needs of the audience.

continues

Table 8–1. *continued*

ELEMENT	UNSATISFACTORY	BASIC	PROFICIENT	DISTINGUISHED
5a: Communicates Effectively *continued*	SLP does not listen carefully to students, parents, and other professionals and fails to provide appropriate clarification when needed. SLP demonstrates inappropriate nonverbal communication style.	SLP may listen to students, parents, and other professionals but often has difficulty providing appropriate clarification when needed. SLP acknowledges the impact of own nonverbal communication style, but usually has difficulty demonstrating this consistently.	SLP listens to students, parents, and other professionals, but may have difficulty providing appropriate clarification when needed. SLP acknowledges the impact of own nonverbal communication style, but may have difficulty demonstrating this consistently.	SLP uses terminology and phrasing consistent with the semantic competence of the audience and includes accurate and complete information, listens carefully to students, parents, and other professionals, takes initiative providing appropriate clarifications when needed, and demonstrates appropriate nonverbal communication style.

ELEMENT	UNSATISFACTORY	BASIC	PROFICIENT	DISTINGUISHED
5b: Writes Reports Clearly and Concisely	SLP does no present information accurately, logically, and concisely. Written reports and letters are inappropriate for the needs of the audience and may include grammatical errors. SLP uses terminology and phrasing inconsistent with the semantic competence of the audience and includes information that is inaccurate and/or incomplete.	SLP intermittently presents information accurately, logically, and concisely. Written reports and letters are sometimes appropriate, using terminology and phrasing often inconsistent with the semantic competency of the audience. SLP sometimes includes information that is accurate and/or complete.	SLP usually presents information accurately, clearly, logically, and concisely. Written reports and letters are appropriate in most situations, using terminology and phrasing consistent with the semantic competency of the audience. SLP usually includes information that is accurate and/or complete.	SLP independently presents written information accurately, clearly, logically, and concisely. Written reports and letters are always appropriate for the needs of the audience. SLP uses terminology and phrasing consistent with the semantic competence of the audience and consistently includes accurate and complete information.

Source: Burlington Edison School District (2010)
http://www.be.wednet.edu/StaffResources/Pathwise/Speech%20Lang%20Path%20Rubric.doc .

Who Are the Stakeholders?

All individuals affected by the practice of speech-language pathology are stakeholders in the effort toward exemplary clinical practice. A competent professional is one who is fully engaged, both professionally and personally, in service delivery. Mentorship can bridge the gap of inspiring new professionals and re-engaging more seasoned clinicians. Mentors may include individuals in leadership positions, co-mentors, and in some cases, self-mentors. There is a component of learning that must take place in order to be a mentor, not just longevity in the workplace.

What Is the Issue?

The improvement and maintenance of clinical services across an array of work sites throughout the career span is one goal of seeking and providing mentorship. The affording of interpersonal growth for all professionals and the prevention of professional fatigue is a second, equally important goal.

Where Can This Take Place?

Mentorship can take many forms and venues. With an open mind, one can be mentored over coffee, over the phone, on the internet, or in many other combinations of communication dialogues and settings. Global mentorship is possible in today's world, as per the article written by Therese Abesamis titled, "A Guiding Hand," in which she describes her mentorship journey from the Philippines to the United States in 2005. The establishment of the ground rules of what one wishes to accomplish and how it can best be done is the next agenda item.

When Does the Process Start?

Mentorship starts with guidance and support necessary to survive and thrive in an increasingly complex and demanding profession.

It requires a careful partnership of an individual or individuals who are well suited to receive the mentorship and mutually benefit. Practitioners may need to be educated about mentorship and what it can offer in order to spark inspiration to engage in the process of mentorship.

Why Engage in Mentorship?

There are as many answers to this question as there are mentoring experiences. Mentorship enhances intrapersonal growth, development, and work-life balance of mentors and mentees alike. Grooming the next generation of professionals is more difficult than it was a generation or two ago when simply recounting interesting anecdotes was the accepted form of teaching and solidifying professional identities. Our audience today is much more diverse. Because of this, their communication styles may be very different than our own, and their backgrounds and experiences sometimes may be greater than our own as well. The expectancies of the new generation of clinicians are much more targeted. Their interest lies in the immediate understanding of practical phenomena and they comprise a wide range of learning styles. They may need education on appreciation of different cultural styles and traditions. It is a two-way street.

How to Engage in This Process?

Whether to include mentorship in one's supervisory practice or whether to seek education on mentorship is a personal decision. There are multiple paths to re-engage in the work setting if one has practiced continuously for many years, such as myself, or whether one has had a break in service or even when one is changing professions. Mentorship is a role that one may take on at any point throughout their career, whether they be a new, mid-career, or seasoned professional. The first step in the process of becoming a mentor is the gathering of information from a meta-mentorship model. It is important to highlight the fact here that the mentorship dyad is highly individualized. A good mentor will try to be uniform in the delivery of his or her core principles, while tailoring their guidance to all of their mentees. It is a sound idea to have a mentorship program that utilizes the substantial resources available from the American Speech-Language Hearing Association (ASHA, 1994, 2007a, 2007b, 2010f). It is equally important to gain a personal perspective of one's goals as a mentor or mentee via individual learning (McCready & Raleigh, 2009). This will maximize the benefit from both personal knowledge and experience, as well as widespread knowledge that has been developed and disseminated in our profession.

Throughout the book, we have paused to consider leadership at different points of professional life. In the field of speech pathology, the role of a supervisor has generally encompassed clinical supervision as well as professional and personal guidance. ASHA has recognized the importance of mentorship in the professional lifespan. In developing and maintaining a rigorous career, it is necessary to refresh and re-engage with other professionals. This is separate from the need of concrete supervision that may take place in the work setting. The following section refers to some of the information that ASHA has put forth in this regard. Although a focus has been placed in evidence gathering for supervision, the development of a rubric for effective mentorship may be more obscure.

The education of a supervisor may be developed both in terms of in-field experience as well as potential mandatory coursework and even eventual certification in this area, should the profession move in this direction. The education and training of a mentor, however, seems to be another matter altogether. ASHA offers rich resources for mentoring at several levels. The S.T.E.P. program (ASHA, 2007b, 2008c, 2009c, 2010a) is the primary source of information and exchange which centers on, and supports, mentorship partnerships. Further information on this program may be obtained at http://www.asha.org/students/gatheringplace/step/default.htm . ASHA also supports the use of the www.mentoring.org website. It is stated by the S.T.E.P. program that mentoring is the second most important variable in professional success after one's education. Mentors help mentees to set goals and reach their goals; help facilitate relationships and opportunities within the profession; and may also help in sustaining jobs and careers. Detailed information is provided by contributing author Andrea Moxley in Chapter 9.

This book has focused on the concept of learning style differences and team-building in increasingly diverse situations. There is a matrix of approaches necessary as opposed to a top-down or bottom-up approach. This approach implies that there are lateral considerations in decision making. The same scenario may have several logical and acceptable responses. Consensus management calls for inclusion of outlying factors as opposed to linear problem solving. An example might be that a given clinical situation may have a different resolution at a different point in time given different transient factors such as timing within the semester, pre-existing situations, and related practical matters.

An effective workplace mentor is one with depth of knowledge and breadth of vision. This person may engage in creative problem solving and help less senior professionals develop similar skills. They do not teach so much as model behavior, which requires an expansive array of interdisciplinary experience. Work experience in different settings and with different management styles may serve as an educational training ground for the mentor. Extensive life and work experience also maximize effective management of oneself and others in all stages of professional and supervisory life.

Some Future Directions in Supervision

When we examine the maturing of this profession, it is important to ask why this is needed and what may be a future direction. The globalization of the workplace in terms of clients, as well as providers and supervisors, is a significant challenge. These challenges extend well beyond the training that was considered adequate when some of the practicing professionals received their education. In some cases, supervisors have extended their training through continuing education. It is a possibility that, in the future, a supervisory fellowship year may be developed, perhaps through distance education modules, in order to standardize the education of supervisors and their discrete professional goals. Mentorship, however, calls on a somewhat different array of skills, the goals of which are different from supervision.

Mentorship in Speech-Language Pathology

As per our accrediting body, ASHA, mentors can assist professionals in a number of ways. The mentor provides access to professional advice, promotes self-confidence, helps the mentee develop new skills, enhances professional opportunity and also assists in job-related stress management in the process. ASHA furthermore provides definitions of key roles in the mentorship process, characteristics of a mentor and mentee, as well as their individual roles. Although the information is geared largely toward the doctoral experience, much of it is directly relevant to the topic at hand. Of particular relevance is the mentoring environment, including aspects which facilitate transition into other settings at the conclusion of mentorship.

It is the premise of the current author that the above information may be extended by looking outside of our immediate profession to other fields in which mentorship is applied and studied. Examples from other helping professions, as well as the for-profit corporate sector, are discussed to look at mentorship through other lenses.

It is essential in today's world, and increasingly in the future, that traditional models of workplace supervision and mentorship be carefully evaluated. Relevance is the key to relating to novice professionals, regardless of their background. Taking cues from industry leaders in unrelated professions may be a helpful strategy. Looking outside of the world of speech-language pathology to the information provided by organizational management may shed light on current concerns in the globalization concept in general.

For example, *The World Is Flat*, by Thomas Friedman (2008) is a best-selling book which describes several key elements that leveled the playing field in the workplace. Such elements include high-speed digital communication devices and availability of search engines. Taken simply, more people are accessing more information more quickly than ever before. Corporate strategies may inspire those in a clinical work setting or private practice. In addition, if one has employees, then one automatically becomes a supervisor or manager. Business people seek to enhance management skills through offering guided mentorship. This guided mentorship may be in the form of management training to convey skills, but also to convey a sense of "organization."

The computer manufacturer IBM has published "The Enterprise of the Future," which compares the new cultural climate to a restless adolescent. Ultimately, this document states that success depends on meeting the needs of imaginative and culturally disruptive phenomena. A desire for change starts with an increase of awareness. Other global giants, such as "World Bank," offer similar educational incentives as basic training, which may also be applied to our profession if we learn and study the models so as to make them applicable to a worldwide consumer base.

Certain speech-language providers are already providing virtual services. If this practice is to thrive, we must respond to compliance and issues beyond our state regulations. Virtual supervision and mentorship already take place with no contact between parties. We must be open to learn, share, and develop new information in order to obtain competence in this arena. Intercultural competence is growing beyond knowing which courtesy is afforded in a particular culture to becoming culturally savvy in a much broader sense. Exposure and education is the key. As such, timeliness is of the essence due to the fact that we are providing services to individuals from all over the world. This is especially true in the metropolitan regions and increasingly in the nonmetropolitan areas. The Medicare Telehealth Enhancement Act of 2009 is aimed at increasing the availability of speech pathology and audiology services in the same vein as the virtual services described above.

Kenneth Staub (2009) writes that multiculturalism is a fact in our society and workplace. Urgent practical and ethical motivations exist for speech-language pathologists engaged in administration and supervision to take responsibility for "cultural fluency." I would add mentors and mentees to this prospective, who also need to respond to the evolving concepts of cultural fluency, for it is a dynamic process. Speech-language pathologists act as conveyors of the culture through increasing communication between individuals. Therefore, we should take leadership in this area in both our organizations and toward one another. Modeling of skills is one way to facilitate behavioral understanding and change, as is active learning. Staub (2009) contributes thoughtful work on how to assess supervisors as multicultural educators, as well as student progression toward competence.

A potential response to this dilemma on how to successfully mentor and supervise speech-language pathologists from an evidence-based approach clearly begins with a review of our existing knowledge and then progresses to a needs analysis within a setting. For this purpose, Dr. Ann Jablon, Chair of the Division of Sciences at Marymount Manhattan College located in metropolitan New York City, contributed an original questionnaire for the purposes of facilitating the mentoring process in a variety of settings (Appendix H). Following is an additional contribution by another Marymount colleague and her student, which consists of a personal narrative on the topic of mentorship for the purposes of this book.

In line with this is the concept of training modules, which may be used as part of a course in clinical supervision and mentorship and/or as an elective in graduate school or postgraduate education. Such offerings currently exist in continuing education programs and encompass the historical issues, current practice, intercultural perspectives, as well as future initiatives. References such as those cited within this book and including the current information would be helpful as initial education on how to teach and supervise the practice of speech-language pathology, as well as how to offer special mentorship to those individuals seeking it.

However, the road to mentorship may not always be a smooth one, even for students and professionals in higher education programs. Sometimes the obstacles are external, others times internal, and most times, a combination of both. This especially may be the case for nontraditional students or clinicians. Educators from many of the allied disciplines have expressed feelings of self-examination at pivotal points in their academic and clinical careers. Journaling or self-assessment through portfolio learning is a way to achieve the personal growth mentorship aims for. It is in this vein that a unique perspective and discussion is offered to illustrate the experience of a successful doctoral student of Hispanic background continuing to seek her professional "place."

Although we are accustomed to working with the needs of bicultural populations as clinicians, the educators of multicultural backgrounds find themselves at a crossroads. The goal no longer is assimilation but a mosaic of intercultural components. The Hispanic culture, of which I am affiliated with, is one of the cultures which has been somewhat underrepresented in the profession due to a myriad of factors (see Carozza, 2002; Roman & Carozza, 2007). This in turn creates the need and desire to answer questions of professional worth. ASHA offers a wealth of information to support the knowledge of culturally and linguistically diverse populations, notably Special Interest Division 14, the Hispanic Caucus, and other documents and resources, The information gained from an individual experience may be just as powerful as the information from a group report. The reader is referred to the following for a first-person account of a mentorship quest that is enlightening in its clarity of expression and which may serve to make the path easier for others to follow. Ms. Vega, who wrote this piece specifically for this book, currently serves as a mentor to several young Latina students in the field of speech-language pathology. Because of my personal interest in issues pertaining to mentorship of minority students, this makes it especially relevant for inclusion in this book.

Latina Mentoring

Blanca E. Vega, Doctoral candidate, Higher and Postsecondary Education Program, Teachers College, Columbia University

"Blanca Vega, I want to be just like you when I grow up!" A recent graduate of my program and future speech pathologist startled me from my story. In the middle of describing to her what I had accomplished within five years of my own college graduation, my young student exclaimed her own desires to work, travel, date, and progress in a career. Even though we did not share similar career paths, I knew what she meant by wanting to be like me—she wanted the same opportunities, maybe travel to the same places, and to date and work before settling into a family and career. A 21-year-old Latina exclaiming to a 34-year-old Latina. I was happy to oblige in a glimpse to her future.

At her age, I did not have a Latina mentor, let alone an Ecuadorian one. Although I will always be grateful to the men and women who have taken me under their wings (even if for a short while) to help me get to my next step, I have always sought The One. The Latina One. The One whose future I can glimpse my naïve eyes through for a look at my own path.

How does one become a Latina mentor without Latino/a mentorship? This question has only crept into my consciousness more fully when asked to describe my experiences as one. Having never really thought through this title in my own life, I had difficulty writing this piece. My own lack of Latina mentorship made my thoughts about myself as a mentor very unclear. Who am I to be a deemed as a Latina mentor? Isn't this a huge responsibility?

That is, until you hear statements like the one my young student made in your presence, of course. The awesome responsibility of it hits like the wind from the train as it rushes past. And after the wind dies down, the work begins.

In this paper, I explore what Latina mentorship has meant in my own life using the narrative of one student who willingly accepted to write about her experience being mentored by me. Using this narrative, I hope to begin exploring the concepts of mentorship and provide one testimonio[1] alongside the many that exist. I will extract important concepts from her narrative and provide a personal analysis of what I have learned from her, the lessons I hope

---

[1]Testimonios, "[are] often seen as a form of expression that comes out of intense repression or struggle . . . " (Latina Feminist Group, p. 13). Additionally, testimonios are stories that disenfranchised people often document and report to "outsiders" to "assert themselves as political subjects to others" (p. 13). Testimonio is a literary genre used in Latin America, particularly by women who share violent political histories. Thus, testimonios can only be shared through individual narratives and report them to "outsiders," encouraging other Latinas to share their stories as well.

to implement in future mentoring relationships, and continue a discussion of what my life has been like without direct Latina mentorship. With this piece, I hope to provide a glimpse into the path of future Latina mentors. In the next section I provide my personal background to help provide context to this evolving story.

Blanca's Story

"A native New Yorker, I am the daughter of Ecuadorian immigrants." This often is how I introduce my work when asked to explore my identity within the context of higher education. In revealing both my U.S. upbringing and my Ecuadorian ancestry, I am fully aware of the position I take as an emerging scholar. This revelation also lies in the center of my work. As a doctoral student in the Higher Education program at Teachers College, I explored the intersection between race and education and its impact on access to and persistence in higher education by students of color. I am particularly interested in the racial stratification of higher education and how this affects Latino students as they move along the academic pipeline. This standpoint is well informed by my own experiences, a kneading of my history, my identity, and the body of knowledge that currently excludes people of color.

At the same time, I also am an administrator for a college. I direct an opportunity program called the Higher Education Opportunity Program (HEOP). HEOP is a state-funded college program that provides access to students who face economic barriers but have demonstrated academic potential. HEOP provides social and economic support to students hoping to attend private independent institutions, such as the one where I currently work. Our students often are the first ones in their families to attend college and few among their friends to progress toward degree attainment. Thus, the program, in addition to providing monetary support, also provides a social support that includes peer relationships and mentorship as well as guidance through the faculty and staff.

As Director of the program, I tend to focus on the matters of politics and administrative work. Nevertheless, I try my very best to stay in close contact with my students. My position allows me to directly mentor students not only for academic purposes but also for professional development. I can also add that my own experiences, which are unique to Latinas and more broadly people of color at predominantly white institutions, allow me to provide a deeper understanding of their college experience. In the next section, I broadly contextualize my experiences as a Latina in academe by providing some data on Latino education.

Background on Latino Education

In 2008, the Latino population comprised 15.4% of the United States population becoming the largest population of color in the country (U.S. Census Bureau, 2010). The Pew Hispanic Center reports that by the year 2020, Latinos will comprise 25% of the U.S. population (Santiago & Brown, 2004). However, Latinos still lag behind other populations in formal education (Fry, 2002; Santiago & Brown, 2004; Schmidt, 2003). The educational disparity of Latinos at all educational levels in comparison to other racial and ethnic groups is at once an economic, social, and political concern (Castellanos, Gloria, & Kamimura, 2006).

Latino students have the lowest enrollment rates and the highest attrition rates throughout the academic pipeline amongst all racial and ethnic groups. Two-thirds of Latinos enroll in college but only 23.2% receive a BA within 10 years of graduating from high school (Swail, Cabrera, Lee, & Williams, 2005). Only 12% of Latinos between the ages of 25 and 29 have attained a college degree (Lopez, 2009). Consequently, Latinos are the least formally educated ethnic group in the United States (Schmidt, 2003). In terms of obtaining a bachelor's degree, Latinas/os lag far behind the overall educational attainment of blacks and whites (Contreras & Gandara, 2006). The view is much bleaker the further one goes through the academic pipeline. Schmidt (2003) writes:

> At the very end of the educational pipeline, Hispanics earn just 4 percent of the doctorates awarded . . . the number of Hispanics earning doctorates or professional degrees actually declined slightly in

recent years . . . Those statistics help explain why Hispanics account for just 2.9 percent of full-time college faculty members and just 3.2 percent of college administrators. (Schmidt, 2003)

Thus, the role of the Latino/a mentor in the educational experiences of young Latinos comes into question in educational research. How is mentoring accomplished when there are so few of us at the end of the pipeline? What is the importance of Latina/o mentorship? In the face of absence, how does the lack of Latino/a mentorship affect the Latino pipeline? In the face of absence, what are the struggles Latino mentors face?

In the next section, I include an excerpt from a student's thoughts on our mentoring relationship. Following this section, I extract important aspects of her description on the importance of mentorship in her life to provide further questions for discussion. Given that this is only one student's understanding with mentorship, it is important to note that this experience cannot capture the full essence of Latino mentorship. Instead, this piece should encourage future research in this area and add a piece to the puzzle of Latino educational attainment.

D's Story

Since I started my college journey at Marymount Manhattan College I have always seen Blanca E. Vega, the Director of the Higher Education program (HEOP), as my mentor. The reason I think of our relationship as a mentoring one is because she is the one person I can always run to when I am struggling in school. Additionally, as my mentor, she has taught me how to deal with racial experiences and how to not let those experiences bring me down. Instead, she teaches me how to take these experiences and enable them to make me a stronger student.

I think one of the main reasons why Blanca and I have formed this mentoring relationship is because I have a lot of respect and admiration for her. She is the first and only Latina woman who I have found in Marymount Manhattan College. She supported me through the transition from high school to college. Finding her made me feel safe and not alone in this transition I was experiencing. Blanca has always been very strict with me, but I have learned that this is because she knows that I am capable of doing more than I am expected and only insists on the best from me.

Blanca plays a very important role in my life. In addition to being my mentor, she is like an older sister. She explains all my options to me, but in the end lets me make the final decision. I believe that this is a very important part of our mentoring relationship. I know that one way for me to grow and take responsibilities is by making my own decisions, and Blanca allows me to do that. I see her as my role model and hope to one day accomplish as many goals as she has. Graduating from college is definitely one of my main goals and with her guidance it has become a much easier process.

Our mentoring relationship began the way most professional relationships are initiated. I got to know Blanca as my mentor and as the Director of the HEOP program. She got to know D as a student. However, as the years have gone by we have built a very strong professional relationship based on trust and communication. Now, Blanca and I even talk about one day working together on a research project. I also have had the opportunity of witnessing various phases in her student life. For example, Blanca passed the first part of her Doctoral exam. I have seeing her sacrifice herself both as a Doctoral student and as the HEOP Director, and she has become great at both jobs.

I am very thankful for having Blanca in my life and do not know how I would have dealt with the college experience if she was not there to guide me. She has become my role model and older sister. One day I hope to accomplish as many goals as she has and to make her proud of all the work I am trying to accomplish. I hope that this mentoring relationship will continue after I graduate from college. I hope to come to her for advice and guidance when in graduate school.

Analysis

The piece written by this student is a beautiful reflection of her development as a student in relation to a mentor. Her testimonio is rich with the importance of mentors in a student's life. From this piece, I have extracted four major themes. They include access to a Latina mentor, knowledge, independence, and vision. I briefly address each theme in the next section.

Access to a Latina Mentor

As noted in my student's testimonio, I was the only Latina staff person who D found at the college. This experience has been recounted among friends who identify as people of color who attended predominantly white institutions. In this absence of more Latino mentors, how do students pick mentors, if at all? Interestingly, she also reports seeing me as an "older sister." To feel like a part of a larger family may be important to certain students, particularly Latino students, who value the role of families in their lives. As an older sister, I am particularly comfortable playing that role, but it is also important to note that I believe there are differences between sister and mentor. Thus, although she views me in this manner, I also have to be conscious of the fact that I am not, and strive to maintain proper boundaries in this respect.

Access to Latina/o mentors in particular fields is also important. The Latino population continues to grow and thus so do their needs. As with my student whom I opened this piece with reminds me, she may view me as a Latina mentor; however, my expertise is in education whereas her knowledge base is beginning to form in the area of speech-language pathology. Perhaps, access to a Latina speech-language pathologist may help this young woman more concretely envision her future in ways that she cannot glimpse through my eyes. Additionally, to address the needs of the growing Latino population, we must be in service to cultivating future professionals in such high needs areas as education and speech pathology.

Knowledge

Being a Latina mentor means that I can speak to a particular experience—that of a Latina in academe who has particular knowledge of what being Latina means in predominantly white institutions. Because this student has dealt with particular instances of racism, it was important for her to speak with someone who has knowledge about handling situations of racism specific to the Latino experience. Although some positions may be created to address this issue specifically, I was not hired to handle this particular phenomenon. My knowledge about college access, persistence, and retention is what I must emphasize in this mentoring relationship. For Latino/a students, their persistence may depend on learning to handle racist experiences. Nevertheless, this added dimension is often easier to discuss with someone who students feel their mentor has direct knowledge of.

Additionally, it is important to gauge just how much information is too much too share. Often, students want to hear more about their mentor's personal life, as is very true in my case. My students, both male and female, will often exclaim, "How come you don't tell me about your personal life and I have to tell you mine?" I remind them that I get paid to listen to them and they do not get paid to listen to me. I also remind them that we have a mentoring relationship and are not peers. I jokingly insist that it would be highly inappropriate for me to discuss my personal relationships with them when I am getting paid to listen to them. As D discusses, she has witnessed some very important parts of my academic career. I may share how I feel about them, but do not dwell in my reality. Instead, I turn it back on her and ask her questions to help her envision her own future.

Ultimately, I believe it is necessary to share information related to the academic life and important for college student development. These kinds of boundaries help them develop their own boundaries as future professionals after college. It is especially important to model this kind of behavior for students who wish to enter such fields as education or counseling, Sharing personal information is knowledge that I choose not to disclose as much, unless of course I feel that it is appropriate for a student to grow and learn from.

Finally, cultivating confidence in students about their own knowledge in their particular field is necessary to help these students see themselves as viable members of their professions. I learned this by working with students who choose different majors than the ones with which I am familiar. For example, my knowledge in the area of speech-language pathology was minimal until I met my students who intend to become speech pathologists. Because I want to understand their passion a little better, I ask them questions about their field, attend their conferences, and try to keep myself updated in this area. My students provide that channel for me and in turn feel that they teach me as well.

Independence

In a mentoring relationship, allowing a student to make her own decisions is highly important. This is the difference between a mentor and an older sister. An older sister (such as myself) may feel strong impulses to tell her younger sisters what to do. As a mentor, however, my job is to provide students with all their options, encourage them to review these carefully, and let them make decisions on their own. Not telling my student exactly what to do, then, is very important. I am sure that if I did tell her what to do, she would *complain* about me being like her older sister and not feel positive about it.

Vision

I believe that my role as a Latina mentor is to help students provide a vision for themselves that they do not see reflected back in media, in their families, or among their peers. As the data show, few Latinos reach beyond the bachelor's degree, a known mechanism toward upward mobility. I believe this can be accomplished by helping students envision for their futures and by seeing them as future colleagues. One of the most impactful statements that a student group advisor made about me in college was how he hoped to see me one day as his future colleague. Before this, I had never realistically thought of myself as a mentor's colleague. By helping students shape their futures, we are telling them that we feel confident that one day we can work collaboratively together and trust the knowledge they acquired. This trust is what ultimately establishes the mentor-mentee relationship, and I strongly believe that this is a value that must be fostered within the Latino academic community.

Conclusion

Sometimes, I wonder if I have received mentoring outside of my fantasies. In other words, I may not have *the latina mentor* that I always dreamed about, who possessed the following qualities: Ecuadorian, global, female, a mother, a daughter, a friend, a researcher, an academic. I dreamed about the day that I would encounter another Ecuadorian woman who would take me under her wing and help me glimpse into my future through her. Instead, in this absence, I have come to know many people- men and women, white and black, who believed in me and encouraged my dreams to become a reality. Thus, I have learned to mentor outside of my fantasies, while I hope to become that fantasy for someone else. Having learned to mentor outside of my fantasies, I believe, although painful, has nevertheless been a very rewarding experience. Learning to become a mentor outside of my fantasies has helped me create different values that *the one* may not have been able to completely accomplish.

As an educational researcher, HEOP provides me with the action part of my research. The activist in me motivates me to persuade students to think beyond a Bachelors degree. Thus, my mentorship toward my students is not only through communication but is also implemented through structure. I provide the structure through which mentorship becomes activated. I do this by providing students with work-study opportunities, formal graduate school exploration, as well as direct one-on-one contact, and I make myself available to students for mentorship. This, I believe is the most important piece in Latina mentorship—providing formal opportunities to Latino students to activate their own knowledge, independence, and vision. My hope is that by doing so, one day they will return the favor by providing other Latinos access to Latino mentorship as well.

How Can Mentorship Be Improved Using an Evidence-Based Approach?

The opportunity to collaborate with my colleagues has provided a great deal of personal and professional insight into my own study of mentorship. In the recent research literature, there has been a merging of interest in the fields of supervision and mentorship, which takes place when supervisors also function as mentors. There is a need for greater reliance on research findings regarding how to broaden our expertise, which is central to the themes contained in this book. There is no doubt that the intrapersonal developmental stage of the supervisor has a tremendous impact on outcomes. Geller and Foley (2009) discuss drawing on input from related fields such as nursing, psychology, social work, and education to better prepare supervisors for their roles as mentors.

Goldstein (2008) also emphasizes that the principle of evidence-based clinical practice may be integrated into clinical supervision using literature review, practice guidelines, and the teaching of systematic review. The latter is most likely the greatest challenge in that substantial attention is given to data gathering, but not necessarily to a critical in-depth assessment and analysis of the research which is at the heart of evidence review. The use of material from fields such as psychology will be valuable in an interdisciplinary perspective on personal growth as a supervisor-mentor. Johnson (2007), in his article, "Transformational Supervision," draws a comparison between academic advisement and supervision that may not entail mentorship. Mentoring-infused supervision, although valuable in developing increasingly reciprocal professional collaborations, requires the considerations of many variables that are not well defined in practice management. Johnson (2007) calls for concerted research into practice skills in this area.

This is an area with which I can concur. Speech-language pathologists will work in a wide variety of workplace settings throughout the course of their career span, have encounters with complex relationships, cultures, and attitudes, and encounter many robust expectations. This is a growing issue in professional supervision and mentorship that is facing many professions, not just speech-language pathology. That issue involves the minority supervisor-mentor and the minority mentee. In my own personal experience spanning over three decades as a certified clinician, I can attest to being the sole minority student with all "traditional" teachers, undergraduate and graduate faculty, clinical supervisors, clinical fellowship year supervisors, as well as departmental supervisors and directors throughout my career. The shift in gender from males to females in the leadership position was also very apparent to me in my own work history.

Eventually, I became the sole Hispanic supervisor of a white female staff at several junctures in my career. I can recall, with pride, my first Latina students and eventual colleagues. This caused me to reach out in ways that were related more to an overidentification on my part to these young professionals. My efforts to mentor them were probably uneven, in the sense that I wanted to "teach them everything I knew" rather than follow a prescribed course in how to supervise. I know better now, and the professions know better now. We have more cross-cultural communication information, leadership strategies, and data regarding best practices in mentorship as well as challenging mentorship cases, such as contained in this book. Nevertheless, this area is still in its infancy.

ASHA is doing a tremendous service to new clinicians who share my background by offering the ASHA S.T.E.P. Program. Andrea "DeeDee" Moxley (contributor) and Melanie Johnson, ASHA S.T.E.P. Mentoring Coaches of the Office of Multicultural Affairs, have been significant sources of information in my effort to learn more about my primary profession as well as its current mentors and mentees. The most recent (2009a) statistics from the ASHA S.T.E.P. office indicate that of 149 mentors, 22 are Hispanic or Latino of varying races. Of the 120 mentees, there are 19 Hispanics. These are impressive gains in attracting and retaining members of one of the most under-represented minorities in our profession.

In addition, as mentioned above, the S.T.E.P. Program provides significant resources via The Gathering Place Mentoring Tips (2004a), sponsored by ASHA. Some of the feedback from mentors and mentees is examined to educate future mentoring teams. The following is an excerpt from an illustrative communication sent by the S.T.E.P. program. It serves to encourage mentors and mentees to seek the input of The Gathering Place Web site, as well as the S.T.E.P. Web site at http://www.asha.org/students/gatheringplace/step.

Does This Sound Familiar?

1. "My mentoring partner was too busy to participate much. It would have been nice if we had more interaction."

2. "My mentee contacted me one time. I responded to the E-mail and didn't hear back. In my opinion, the mentee should be seeking out the mentor initially and on an ongoing basis."

3. "My mentee pretty much always fizzled out. I didn't think I should hound them with e-mails. If they didn't respond after several E-mails, I let it go."

4. "I think perhaps we needed a better introduction to each other and some ideas on how we should work together."

Source: E-mail communication to the author received Jan. 2010.

Of the above quotes, the one that stands out in terms of the current chapter is number 4. If we examine the statement we see two issues. The first issue being the importance of the introduction to the mentoring process and the second being the need for a "road map" of how to proceed. These issues are even more critical, perhaps with newer mentors and mentees, as well as those from nontraditional backgrounds in which the mentorship culture is not as well defined.

As the trend to seek bilingual and bicultural speech-language pathologists to treat the growing number of bilingual and bicultural speakers continues, the need for mentorship will continue to grow. If there were prementorship initiatives reaching down to the high school level, the candidates for entry into our profession would increase. Recent research conducted by the author for the purposes of this book revealed that the Hispanic Scholarship Consortium had 10 awardees in 2009 to 2010, nine females and one male.

One of the recipients, a student at the University of Texas in Austin, has chosen speech-language pathology as her area of academic concentration. (See http://www.hispanicscholar.org for further details.) In this manner, the profession "primes the pump" for future minority clinicians and faculty as well as supervisors and mentors. This is of considerable importance in terms of access to the profession and facilitating future clinicians beyond the initial point of entry into the profession, which is critical for students of all backgrounds!

Mentorship has many forms. As a more mature professional, I attempted mentorship for more advanced goals. However, I was not able to attain a mentor with a suitable background primarily due to age and experience in the profession. Instead, it may have been more appropriate for me to seek a peer mentor. This is important because mentoring needs do not exist only at the earlier career stages but may exist at other significant junctures as well. A suggested paradigm might include steps such as the following.

Mentor trainees develop a reflective statement and are certified as trainers for next cycle of mentors via:

1. Mentors read accrued information about outcomes from prior dyads

2. Mentors select an article from leadership literature to present

3. Mentors report on mentorship accomplishments at conclusion of training

A Road Map

Rather than initiating professional concerns at the first meeting, a social meeting with sharing of personal-professional information and goals may be conducive to setting the stage for good mentorship. A second meeting could be used to establish mentee, mentor, and program goals for purposes of "establishing" the contract. Mutual assignments are agreed on, as well as terms of communication such as how often and in what form (i.e., E-mail, face-to-face). A visual framework, such as charting progress, can support the mentoring relationship by establishing a mentorship by objectives chart. This may include timeliness of assignments, number of parent and client interactions, and other quantifiable data. Weekly and monthly reviews of progress should be recorded for the purposes of final report and outcome success, depending on the time frame of the clinical setting.

Simultaneously, the supervisor may consider obtaining outside supervision in the form of individual or group mentorship meetings. A senior mentor would discuss types of mentorship, how-to's and how-not's, conducting role-play scenarios, presentation of video practice, assistance in conversational dyads, and teaching other helpful strategies. Informal and original material may be used for these purposes, as well as curriculum based on professional resources, such as this book and others. At times, it may be necessary for the senior mentor to participate in the first meeting and at regular intervals as well as at specific junctures in order to train the junior mentor(s). The senior mentor may bring in all supervisors for focus groups, conduct debriefings of mentors at end of training, as well as maintaining a database of agreed on manageable outcomes. These may include databases of communicative effectiveness and satisfaction ratings by the mentor and the student clinician.

The whole purpose of this is independent problem-solving at either level, examination of results of a designated objective, collaboration and information sharing, and the ability to seek mentorship appropriately regardless of level in one's career. The ability to provide and use resources may be accomplished in all of these levels as one moves along the continuum.

This chapter explored what it means to be a mentor, where one can go for further resources and guidelines to improve mentoring skills, what is at stake for everyone involved in the mentoring process, as well as the need for mentorship in minority populations. Although the scope of this book does not cover any of these topics fully in depth, it is important for young professionals entering this field to be aware of everything that the role of supervisor/mentor entails, as well as what to expect.

What's Next?

The issue of mentoring is further explored in the following chapter, which addresses some of the different types of mentoring and some current mentoring programs.

CHAPTER 9

A Model of Mentorship: Expert Practice

Mentoring can provide insight that is "outside of our day-to-day life." The role of a mentor is to serve as a coach, a source of encouragement, a resource, a champion, and devil's advocate.

American Speech-Language-Hearing Association, n.d.(a)

Overview

Mentoring can be used to connect students to their intended area of clinical practice. In a study conducted in the United Kingdom, nursing students were matched to mentors on the basis of area of clinical expertise. Results from follow-up surveys indicated that students felt more "connectedness with the clinical area" based on their mentoring experience (Mysall, Levitt-Jones, & Lathlean, 2008, p. 1840).

Mentoring also may be used to provide mentees with solutions to real-life practicum issues. In a study that connected practicum teachers to mentors in an online mentoring program, students reported that the online mentoring experience enhanced their ability to solve real-life classroom discipline issues in real time (Hew & Knapczyk, 2007, p. 31).

Mentoring provides the opportunity for mentees and mentors to freely and safely communicate frustrations about their current work environment. In a study conducted by Simonsen, Luebeck, and Bice (2009), the authors matched beginning science and mathematics teachers in order to provide content-based mentoring via computer-mediated communication. Feedback from participants identified one benefit of mentoring: It serves as a private opportunity to communicate, share ideas and discuss frustrations with administrators, colleagues, and parents (Simonsen, Luebeck, & Bice, 2009, p. 66).

E-mentoring, or online mentoring, provides the platform to reach a broad base of participants. The ability to remotely connect mentee to mentor can provide a variety of successful outcomes. The American Speech-Language-Hearing Association (ASHA) first initiated an E-mentoring program as a component to the Minority Student Leadership program. The success of this E-mentoring component led to the inception of the ASHA Gathering Place in 2004 to reach a broader base of participants. The ASHA Gathering Place is the mentoring portal that holds ASHA's mentoring programs. ASHA Membership Program Manager Melanie Johnson and the Office of Multicultural Affairs collaborated to develop the ASHA Gathering Place and its first mentoring program, the Student to Empowered Professional (S.T.E.P.) 1:1 mentoring program. ASHA developed the S.T.E.P. program as part of a collaborative effort to develop a tool for recruitment/retention efforts aimed at helping historically underrepresented populations in the field of communication sciences and disorders (CSD). In this chapter, we explain how ASHA used data to develop and enhance the ASHA S.T.E.P. mentoring program.

According to ASHA 2009 year-end counts (ASHA, 2009a), approximately 6.9% of ASHA members, nonmember certificate holders, and international affiliates are members of a racial minority [compared with 24.9% of the U.S. population according to the 2000 Census (Grieco & Cassidy, 2001)], including 1.3% who have self-identified as multiracial (compared with 2.4% of the U.S. population). Additionally, 3.7% identified their ethnicity as Hispanic or Latino, compared with 12.5% of the U.S. population. It is important that the goal of your mentoring program support the overall mission or vision. The goals of the S.T.E.P. program are to:

■ connect self-motivated students with experienced mentors in meaningful, one-to-one mentoring relationships;

■ support mentoring relationships through guided learning experiences;

■ provide online resources for all students and mentors seeking tools, information, and inspiration;

■ facilitate the continued recruitment and retention of racial/ethnic minority students.

A clearly defined, measurable goal will assist you in establishing objectives, benchmarks, or measures. In the S.T.E.P. program, objectives and benchmarks of success were determined based on the program goals. Short-term objectives measure the number of participants in the mentoring program and the number of participants satisfied with the mentoring process. Long-term objectives track the mentees' trajectory from students to ASHA-certified members and the volunteerism of mentors in the Association. Measures include data collected from enrollment forms, surveys, and contact tracking. The long-term objective for the S.T.E.P. mentoring program is to support the association's efforts for the recruitment and retention of historically underrepresented populations in communication sciences and disorders. This clearly defined objective established our pool of potential mentees as historically underrepresented populations.

Some additional potential mentees could be:

■ undergraduate students;

■ Ph.D. students;

■ nontraditional students;

■ bilingual students;

■ international students;

■ new professionals in the field;

■ new faculty;

■ professionals transitioning from one area of the field to another;

■ professionals reentering the field.

It is equally important to consider the potential mentor pool. The mentors should possess those desired areas of expertise and experience detailed previously. Some examples of potential mentors could include:

■ current or former master's-level students;

■ current or former doctoral students with or without a research focus;

■ junior- or senior-level faculty;

■ content area experts;

■ bilingual service providers;

■ leaders or volunteers in the field;

■ researchers;

■ presenters;

■ writers;

■ retirees.

There should be a significant discussion surrounding the selection of potential mentoring pools. Mentors could have a lot to offer; however, it is essential that the selecting organization know what the mentor has to offer the mentee—for example, clinical expertise, information about clinical setting, perspective on establishing a research lab, or sharing guidance on how to get through an academic program. These desired characteristics will become matching criteria for your mentoring program. These matching criteria drove the development questions on the S.T.E.P. enrollment form (Appendix I). We also collect demographic data, including race, gender, and ethnicity, to address the primary long-term objective of recruitment and retention of underrepresented populations. In addition, we asked questions to determine the success of program marketing venues and future considerations for the development of the program (e.g., "Would you accept text messages?"). Former questions asking participants if they were on Facebook led to the development of the ASHA S.T.E.P. Mentoring Program fan page and the ASHAStep Twitter account.

The S.T.E.P. mentoring coaches determined that the matching criteria would be based on the mentees' desired area of expertise, intended work setting, intended primary work function, intended clinical age population, and language(s) spoken. S.T.E.P. mentees were also asked to describe their career goals. The mentor and mentee with the most number of common responses were matched; however, responses to the mentees' career goals were carefully considered, as well. At times, a mentee would indicate one area of expertise, such as autism, but the career goal would state that he or she was interested in establishing a private practice. The desired mentor match would then become individuals with a private practice first, regardless of whether autism was a primary area of expertise. This open-ended career goal response has become pivotal to the matching process.

Matching criteria are determined based on program goals and objectives. For example, the primary focus for the S.T.E.P. program is to match based on areas of clinical expertise. It is important to gather feedback on the effectiveness of the program's matching criteria. We invited mentors and mentees from 2006 to 2007 to provide input to help ASHA confirm that the appropriate criteria was being used in the 2007 S.T.E.P. Program Evaluation Report (ASHA, 2008c). Of the 304 individuals invited, 131 chose to respond to this survey. Mentors and mentees were asked to rate the level of importance of each of the potential matching criterion. Table 9–1 combines the ratings of "very important" and "important" to each of the potential criteria in order of highest to lowest.

Respondents were provided the opportunity to write in additional criteria. A number of participants wrote "geographic location." This potential criterion was added as to the list of desired criteria beginning in 2008. Location is not a primary consideration;

Table 9–1. Combined Percentage of Responses of "Important" and "Very Important"

Potential matching criteria	% of "important" and "very important" responses
Area of expertise	79%
Work setting	73%
Primary work function	73%
Age of population served	70%
Language(s) spoken	66%
Race/ethnicity	33%
Gender	19%

however, if there are two mentors of equal value in terms of area of expertise and work setting, location becomes the deciding factor. For mentees who are bilingual or who would like to be bilingual service providers, language(s) spoken becomes the most important criterion.

Feedback by program participants consistently underscores the importance of matching and of the criteria for doing so. The perceived success of a mentoring program often rests in the success of the match. Feedback in a 2008 S.T.E.P. Year-End Survey reported, "It would be helpful to better match those being mentored with mentors who work in their potential or desired specialty. For instance, I research adult language but was placed with a professor whose studies focus on child language. She was helpful and kind, but it may have been more fruitful for me to have been matched with a similar mind." Identifying the target population will provide the basis for determining the elements of the mentoring program, including E-mentoring components, establishing the time line, establishing the budget, and developing the marketing plan.

E-mentoring components. The Web provides an excellent platform to establish and deliver a mentoring program. A Web page can serve as a central location for enrollment forms, program information, and resources. Additional components to consider include the number of social media outlets—such as Skype, Twitter, Facebook, and LinkedIn—that will allow the mentor and mentee to E-network. Mobile phones and texting can also serve as a potential source of program support.

It is important to have resources available on mentoring and on successful mentoring relationships. Be sure to emphasize the importance of communication and the value of discussing goals. If you can, establish a Web site or Web page, which serves as a good central location. Having a strong Web presence allows you to brand your program and to serve as a warehouse for information. The 2008 S.T.E.P. Program Evaluation Report (ASHA, 2009c) was sent to 338 invited mentors and mentees. Fifty-two individuals responded to the question asking about E-mail and newsletter topics. Responses included:

- professional goals and goal setting;
- resume writing, as it pertains to specific job settings;
- grants and scholarships;
- re-entry into the field and training in other areas;
- time management;
- financial aid;
- advice on how to motivate mentor–mentee interaction;
- starting your new career;
- men in the professions;
- questions to ask during a clinical forum or interview;
- do's and don'ts for setting up a practicum;
- common pitfalls of new clinicians;

■ leadership development in the professions;

■ publication opportunities.

ASHA carefully considers mentors' and mentees' responses as we further develop resources for placement on the web. We also may use these responses to create E-mail messages that are sent to future program participants.

Time frame. It is important to establish a reasonable timeframe for the mentoring commitment. Other factors to consider are:

■ Staff resources.

■ Intended recruitment period.

■ Most beneficial timeframe for your participants' goals. This timeframe might include calendar time (e.g., holidays/seasonal), academic time (if individuals are students or professors), and transitional times (e.g., new year's resolutions, back-to-school prep)

For consistency, it is important to maintain a similar enrollment period from year to year. However, remember to monitor the completion of the enrollment forms. If all of them come in after your deadline, then the dates might need to be modified. The enrollment period can be established once you set the target population.

Budget. Budget and staff allocation are also important elements to a mentoring program. Remember that you might not see an immediate return on investment for a fledgling mentoring program. Budgetary considerations include the cost of any direct mailings for marketing and program giveaways; E-mail blasts are reasonable solutions that can help you save money (especially regarding postal costs). Staff allocation and resources are a significant indirect cost for any mentoring program. And don't underestimate the Web as a valuable networking tool: It's a great low-cost way to connect participants to all kinds of helpful resources.

Marketing plan. A wise marketing move is to use all available resources to connect mentors with mentees and to advertise your program. Low-cost ways include E-mail blasts, list serves, and placing information on the Web site to get the program out. Data collection from enrollment forms show that placement of the program on the Web and E-mail blasts are the most effective way for mentees to receive information about the S.T.E.P. mentoring program. ASHA has collected (via the ASHA S.T.E.P. Mentoring Enrollment Form) data over the years on "how you heard about the program." Table 9–2 indicates the responses from mentees and mentors to these questions for the programs beginning in the fall of 2006, 2007, 2008, and 2009. More than one response was allowed in the 2006 program and responses were not required for the 2006 program. Shaded boxes indicate questions that were not asked. Data collected indicate that E-blasts and placement on the Web site are the most effective ways of communicating with mentors.

Direct mailing with an appeal from the association president is effective for recruiting mentors but is not necessarily the most cost-effective marketing method. Again, coordinators of a mentoring program must consider the target population. Mobile phone devices and texting offer the potential to use text messages to recruit mentors and mentees. However, at this time, texts can incur pay-per-view costs. Potential participants may be discouraged or put off if they must pay to see the recruitment message. Do not overextend the invitation to either a mentor or mentee pool, or else you may end up with too many mentees or too many mentors. It is more important to have an overabundance of mentors than mentees. This gives you the opportunity to maximize the match by selecting the mentor who will be most well-suited for each mentee based on the mentee's specified areas of interest. During the recruitment period, one recommended practice is to monitor how many applications you received. This will help you understand which population to focus on in your additional recruitment efforts. Whether you will receive more mentors or mentees is not easily predicted. Recently, ASHA has used Facebook and Twitter to advertise the program. Data are tracked so that ASHA can determine whether any participants have heard about our program via social media outlets.

Table 9–2. How Mentors and Mentees Heard About the S.T.E.P. Program

	Mentees 2006 (not required)	Mentors 2006 (not required)	Mentees 2007	Mentors 2007	Mentees 2008	Mentors 2008	Mentees 2009	Mentors 2009
I received an E-mail	*56%	*10%	39.4%	73.6%	45.2%	84.2%	40.4%	70.3%
At a meeting		*0%	1.1%	0%	2.2%	0.3%	0%	0%
From my college professor	*36%		6.7%		6.7%		2.2%	
From my program director	*10%		1.7%		0.7%		0%	
From the NSSLHA Web site	*8%		17.8%		11.9%		0%	
I read about it in ASHA Leader	*4%	*40%	2.2%	7.1%	1.5%	4.1%	2.2%	6.2%
I read about it in NSSLHA News and Notes	*6%		2.2%		0.7%		13.5%	
I read about it on the ASHA Web site	*8%	*10%	18.3%	10.8%	23.0%	7.4%	24.7%	16.6%
Other	*10%	*30%	8.3%	3.3%	7.4%	2.5%	12.4%	2.1%
Through on-line social network (e.g., MySpace, Facebook, etc.)					0.7%	0.3%	4.5%	0.7%
I received a letter	*30%		2.2%	3.8%		0.5%		0.7%
From a colleague		*0%	1.4%		0.8%		3.4%	

Communication. The frequency of communication can be difficult to balance. Responses to questions about program communication on program evaluation reports have provided inconsistent information. Responses from participants typically range from "not enough communication" to "just the right amount" to "too much communication." Certain E-mail messages might be vital to the program, so cutting them will not be an option. Granted, it is not likely that the success of the program will be based solely on frequency of communication; however, it can enhance the participants' experience. One suggestion is to reserve E-mail use to only the most pressing, pertinent messages about the program.[1] Social media outlets provide a good way to connect mentors and mentees to messages relevant to mentoring and the CSD field.

Communication to the S.T.E.P. Mentoring program is tracked. Beginning in Fall 2006, contacts were tracked by participant, mentor, and mentee.

- 2005–2006 program—211 contacts tracked

- 2006–2007 program—78 contacts tracked (47 from mentors and 31 from mentees)

- 2007–2008 program—44 contacts tracked (29 from mentors and 14 from mentees)

- 2008–2009 program—58 contacts tracked (43 from mentors and 15 from mentees)

- 2009–2010 program—25 contacts tracked (21 from mentors and 4 from mentees)

ASHA has noted a steady decline in contacts from participants over the years. Reasons for this decline could include the development of Web resources and use of technology, including E-mail and

---

[1]*Note:* Recent reports indicate that spam blockers and firewalls may prevent you from communicating via E-mail with some of your participants. Be sure to include your name, telephone number, address, E-mail address, and Web site in the message. This will help ensure that your message will get through some of the security mechanisms on the Web.

social media. The 211 contacts tracked in 2005 to 2006 program led to the development of E-resources, including the ASHA Gathering Place Mentoring Manual (ASHA, 2004a). The majority of questions from ASHA mentors and mentees tend to center around how to establish a mentoring relationship. These questions led to the establishment of two web discussion boards, Mentoring 101 and Starting a Successful Mentoring Relationship. These 1-hour events featured former participants and S.T.E.P. mentoring coaches answering mentors' and mentees' questions "live." These events are archived on the ASHA Web site so that future participants can read questions and responses from individuals who have already experienced the S.T.E.P. mentoring program (see Appendix J). Web forum events or chats can provide low-cost ways to reach a broad target audience.

Surveys. Online surveying programs, such as Survey Monkey, can provide low-cost opportunities to survey the mentors and mentees already enrolled in your mentoring program. Surveys should be conducted twice during the mentoring session. The first survey should be conducted midway through the mentoring program; this allows you to check in with participants to determine on how things are going) and to resolve any issues or problems before the end of the session. The second survey should be conducted at the end of the mentoring year; this allows you to ask questions that will help you measure your benchmarks. Benchmarks should relate back to the program objectives and should be used to determine any modifications that need to be made. Any mentoring program should have a benchmark determining the participants' perceived success of the mentoring program. S.T.E.P. mentoring program midpoint surveys are informal E-mail messages that do not require a response. Participants are asked if they have been communicating and if they need any additional assistance. Beginning in 2007, ASHA began inviting mentors and mentees to participate in a formal year-end survey for the S.T.E.P. program, examining the quality of the program (Appendix D).

Each year, mentees are asked how successful they feel they were at accomplishing the goals that were set for this program. Table 9–3 indicates the combined ratings of "successful" and "very

Table 9–3. Combined Percentages of "Successful" and "Very Successful"

S.T.E.P. Program Evaluation Report	% of "successful" and "very successful" ratings
2007	30%
2008	49%
2009	64%
2010	70%

successful" in response to questions in S.T.E.P. Program Evaluation Reports 2007 to 2010.

ASHA uses these results to craft (and modify, if necessary) additional information on the importance of establishing goals for the S.T.E.P. mentoring program. This information is sent to mentors and mentees several times during the onset of the program. The process is as follows: After mentees fill out and send in the enrollment form, ASHA sends them additional information. Later on, the E-mail containing notification of the mentor match contains information about setting a goal for the program with a link to the "Writing Goals and Objectives" form on the ASHA Web site (ASHA, n.d.[b]) The mentor is also copied on this information so that he or she can assist mentees in establishing program goals.

Coordinators of the mentoring program may establish benchmarks that evaluate data to be measured over time. The primary goal of the S.T.E.P. mentoring program is for mentees to become ASHA-certified members. You cannot measure the success of this goal only at the end of a program cycle; rather, you must track the participants' trajectory as they proceed through the program. However, the percentage of S.T.E.P. mentees becoming ASHA-certified members can be determined by tracking them over their academic career. Seventy-nine of the 85 mentees in the 2004 to 2005 S.T.E.P. program were listed in the ASHA member database. Eighty percent of ASHA S.T.E.P. mentees from the initial 2004 to 2005 program have become ASHA-certified members. It is important also to consider those 20% of mentees who did not become ASHA-certified members. There are a number of contributing factors that might be of interest. Mentees may have changed career paths, transferred academic programs, experienced difficulty with the PRAXIS, or were unable to get through the clinical practicum. Examination of these factors might significantly assist in changing the number of mentees who become ASHA-certified members.

Future Program Developments

The increasing prevalence of social media has created myriad possibilities for mentoring in the CSD field. The ease, speed, and accessibility of technologic advances in communication—such as social networking sites, blogs, E-mail blasts, and so forth—provide new ways of interacting professionally, eliminating former barriers such as geographic location, distance, and time (and often, saving money in the process). Social media provides countless opportunities to communicate and to create communities within your mentoring program. Mentoring can become "e-mentoring" and networking can become "e-networking" using some of these tools.

Blogging is a great way to provide mentees with a peek into what the daily workload and/or issues might be like. You could have a large number of followers/mentees for only one mentor blogger. A name draw might be one successful way to give career changers, students, or individuals looking to change their work setting a glimpse at a specific job. It also could be a good way to highlight academic careers.

In Fall 2009, the ASHA S.T.E.P. Mentoring Program started Twitter and Facebook components. Facebook is an online social entity that allows individuals to become "friends." Friends may share wall posts about day-to-day life, photos, and videos. The Facebook page for the ASHA S.T.E.P. Mentoring program has 93 fans. Information is posted about successful mentoring relationships and interesting news related to the CSD professions. There has been minimal posting on the discussion board about clinical forum experiences.

The ASHA S.T.E.P. Mentoring Program on Twitter has 55 followers. Twitter allows you 140 character spaces to communicate a message. Even if you are not on Twitter, you might wish to search on some common CSD terms to see what people are talking about. This can be an informal way to gather data about what your audience is talking about and needs. A Twitter account can be linked to a Facebook account, so postings made on Facebook would automatically post to Twitter (and vice versa). "Hash tags" allow you to focus your tweets on an individual event. For example, "#ASHA09" would mean that you are trying to talk about the ASHA '09 event. This is great when you are trying to encourage candid, up-to-the-minute chatter.

The 2009 S.T.E.P. Program Evaluation (ASHA, 2010a) asked mentees about participation on Facebook and ideas for future Facebook discussions or Tweets. Twenty-seven of the 115 invited mentees indicated 100% participation on Facebook, 11% participation on Twitter, 7% participation on LinkedIn, and 11% on other social media outlets.

Eight participants reported the following topic ideas for future Facebook discussion or Tweets (these ideas will be vetted for consideration in future programs):

- informal discussions among all mentors/mentees regarding the STEP program
- scholarships (especially for older students)
- graduate school resources
- GRE/MAT exam prep
- nontraditional students' guide to success in speech-language pathology/audiology programs
- starting your own private practice
- multicultural-related discussions
- travel-abroad opportunities

■ intervention research

■ neurogenic disorders

■ a question-and-answer forum with other speech-language pathologists

■ clinical training

Year-end surveys report consistent feedback from participants about the inability to meet a mentor or mentee in person. Videoconferencing tools, such as Skype, provide users with the opportunity to meet "face-to-face" virtually.

The ASHA S.T.E.P. Mentoring program uses a number of forms and surveys to collect data that assist in program evaluation. Mentors' and mentees' responses to these forms and surveys can assist ASHA in future program development; however, these responses do not necessarily measure the value of mentoring. The following testimonials serve as a reminder of the power of mentoring in a career.

> *I have served as a mentor to hundreds of students and young professionals during the 37 years of my career. My role is that of coach as well as cheerleader. Through guidance, encouragement, nagging, pushing, and sometimes scolding, the protégé can ascend to much greater heights than he/she thought possible.* Gloria Weddington (2006)

> *My greatest sense of satisfaction as a mentor comes when former mentees become mentors. . . . Mentoring is truly continuing the cycle of care through life's journey. It is one of the greatest responsibilities and joys of professional life.* Dolores Battle (2007)

> *My S.T.E.P. mentor has been my personal sounding board, advice source, and saving grace.* Aly Rivero (Quevedo, 2007)

This chapter looked at mentoring in the 21st century, and explored some of the technologic advances that have contributed to more modern, up-to-date mentoring forms and programs. It is important that we keep up-to-date with current trends and applications of technology as a means by which to keep our practice current and relevant. This chapter also discussed one of ASHA's recent undertakings, the S.T.E.P. program, aimed at empowering students from racial/ethnic minority backgrounds enrolled in the field of speech-language pathology.

What's Next?

Having spent a great deal of time examining the past research, issues and challenges, and possible solutions, it is now time to look ahead toward the future. As such, the following chapter looks at some future directions for clinical supervision.

SECTION III

Creating Supportive Contexts for Supervision and Mentorship

CHAPTER 10

Learning from Experience: Future Directions for Clinical Supervision

One mark of a great educator is the ability to lead students out to new places where even the educator has never been.

Thomas Groome

Traditionally, supervision research and practice has maintained a predisposition toward conceptualizing clinical supervision as a strictly pedagogical process (such as Glaser & Donnelly's 1989 work on data-based supervision methods) and often from positivistic paradigms in which knowledge is external to the supervisee. Inherent in this traditional view is the perspective that the supervisor's role is primarily one of information provider. Geller and Foley (2009) described traditional themes in supervision as including: "(a) an emphasis on discipline-specific knowledge; (b) an instructional, didactic, and information approach to supervision; (c) minimal attention to the centrality of relationships in all learning environments; and (d) less emphasis on the internal, affective, and intersubjective dimensions of relationships" (p. 23). Future directions in supervision practice may include viewing the supervisory process as a constructivist, facilitative process through which *adults* learn in a *workplace* context through experience. In fact, recent thoughts on supervision (such as the recent work of Geller & Foley and Fitzgerald, 2009 among others) include multimodal foci and perspectives (supervisor and supervisee) which favor learning by affective, relationship-based means *in addition* to more traditional cognitive-based approaches. It is apparent from the burgeoning evolution of supervision approaches that the theoretical bases of supervision are expanding to include whole person learning perspectives, although from a pedagogic perspective.

This chapter aims to provide a future direction for research in and practice of clinical supervision in speech-language pathology. The future of clinical supervision will likely include a multitude of considerations beyond cognitive learning strategies when working with supervisees. This chapter posits that adult education models, especially those which directly deal with learning from experience, have much to offer by way of directing research efforts and practice in clinical supervision. Implicit in this direction is the introduction of constructivist views of reality in which knowledge is viewed as arising from the person versus existing outside the human. By attempting to balance the discipline-specific information with the necessary individual processes which must take place for clinical learning to occur in meaningful ways, it is hoped this additive approach will lead to more fruitful research and practice in supervision.

Clinical supervision is not unique to the field of speech-language pathology and a wide variety of approaches and models are available to the supervisor from multiple fields (Clifford, Macy, Albi, et al., 2005; Cogan, 1973; Lambie & Sias, 2009; Walsh, Nicholson, Keough, et al., 2003; Winstanley & White, 2003). What has been missing, however, is a conceptualization of supervision as consisting of the development of an adult to function in a workplace. Although academic preparation consists of its own flux of approaches to teaching and authentic contexts related to course material, supervision of the student, the clinical fellow, or the novice clinician is based on the premise that independent practice of speech-language pathology requires actual performance of work in an authentic context. Implicit in supervision is a real-world context that requires immediate application of theory, ideas, inclinations, and beliefs. The presence of this real world context is mutually beneficial to the clinical supervisor and the supervisee in that the focus of the process is client-driven, that is, the purpose of practice is to meet the client's needs. This authentic context provides the necessary experience a supervisee requires to develop into an independent practitioner. This is in stark contrast to traditional academic preparation where ideas are presented and discussed in classrooms, often void of authentic context for application of concepts. Furthermore, the context of clinical supervision is real. Pedagogic approaches to experiential learning which consist of role-play and simulations, whereas appropriate for classroom-based activities, lack the presence of a real client with real emotions and needs. This authentic context may be leveraged to enhance supervisees' clinical learning if the natural splendor of the clinical context is adequately utilized.

Andragogy

In realizing clinical supervision in speech-language pathology as a process whereby adults are developed in an authentic workplace context, it is vital to view a supervisee's development as a process of learning through experience. It also is necessary to view the supervisee as an adult learner with different needs and learning behaviors than one would expect of a child. As Rowden (2007) pointed out, "Adults are not just big children—after all" (p. 41). In traditional pedagogic views, the supervisor was seen as an all-knowing expert whose sole role in supervision was passing on her knowledge to the supervisee. This orientation, however, has changed. Additive to the burgeoning multi-modal approaches is a more adult-oriented approach to clinical supervision, what Knowles (1970) termed *andragogy*.

Andragogy, as Knowles conceptualized it, came to consist of six assumptions regarding adults and their learning: (1) First, adults are self-directed in their learning. (2) Adults enter the learning situation with vast and varied past experience when compared to younger learners. This past experience acts as a lens through which new experiences are perceived. (3) Adults require some impetus to trigger a need to know. This assumption about adult learners is in direct opposition to the more traditional pedagogic approaches to supervision in which the supervisor possesses the most social power in the clinical learning situation and effectively decides what the supervisee should learn and how he/she should learn it. (4) Similarly, adults approach learning situations with a task-centered point of reference. Adults tend to learn what is necessary to effectively deal with the clinical situation at hand versus a pre-programmed curriculum devised by the supervisor. (5) Adults' motivations to learn come from both intrinsic and extrinsic sources. Whereas the student is seen in a traditional sense to be motivated by grades (extrinsic motivation), adults are strongly motivated by intrinsic forces, such as becoming a competent practitioner (Rowden, 2007). Extrinsic motivators, however, also play a role in adult learning. In the clinical supervision situation, extrinsic motivation to learn may indeed involve receiving a passing grade in the practicum or a promotion to senior clinician for those who have completed their graduate training. (6) Lastly, adults require an understanding of why they should learn something. In a supervision experience, it is much more likely a supervisee will actively approach a learning situation if he/she knows why learning a concept is important to clinical practice in speech-language pathology. This is opposed to only knowing that she has to understand a concept in order to appease the supervisor (Knowles, 1970; Knowles, Holton III, & Swanson, 2005).

Although these assumptions regarding adult learning could be applied to children as well, it is clear that adults require a stake in the learning process to effectively and efficiently learn about work. Using these assumptions about adult learning, however, requires that the supervisor rethink traditional models and approaches to clinical supervision. Luckily, there is a rich research literature regarding humans' abilities and proclivities to learn through experience. These scholarly works may lead the theory and practice of clinical supervision into new, uncharted territory in the future.

Experiential Learning Theory

Kolb and Kolb (2005) outlined six propositions of experiential learning theory based on the work of prominent scholars in education. Taken together, these propositions may lead clinical supervision into new territories with learning from experience forming the conceptual framework for meaningful action in the learning-centered workplace.

Proposition One

"Learning is best conceived as a process, not in terms of outcomes" (p. 194). When clinical supervision is viewed in this light, the act of supervising (and being supervised) is focused on the process through which learning occurs rather than the result of the supervision process. Rather than solely analyzing the supervisee's behavior with a client, a focus on process would attend more readily to how the supervisee reached the conclusion regarding how he/she would behave with a client.

More specifically, what resources were accessed and which learning strategies did the supervisee implement to reach his/her decision regarding this client? A focus on process versus outcome may better prepare the supervisee for the myriad nonroutine conditions she is likely to encounter in the workplace in the future. Developing the intrapersonal skills to successfully navigate the workplace learning environment early on likely will lead to better clinical decisions when the level of supervision is reduced or is absent altogether.

Proposition Two

"All learning is relearning" (p. 194). The clinical learning process is development and refinement of what is already known. Bringing the supervisee's beliefs and ideas about the clinical process to the surface in order to critique and refine them is at the core of learning from experience. Facilitating a novice clinician's ability to be critical of her own ideas regarding clinical practice and to improve upon these ideas as time and varied clinical experiences transpire will further prepare him/her to make sound decisions independently in the future.

Proposition Three

"Learning requires the resolution of conflicts between dialectically opposed modes of adaptation to the world" (p. 194). Learning is a struggle between what one knows and what one perceives. In order for clinical learning to occur, a disconnect between what the supervisee thought was correct and what he/she is seeing, hearing, thinking, or feeling in the clinical situation is necessary. This dissonance between what one believes and the current workplace situation is necessary and a prerequisite to "relearning" (see Proposition Two above).

Proposition Four

"Learning is a holistic process of adaptation to the world" (p. 194). It is known that learning requires more than simply relying on cognition and its varied processes (Merriam, Caffarella, & Baumgartner, 2007). Learning is a function of one's thinking, feeling, behaving, and perception. Although recent scholarly developments in clinical supervision have begun to explore the role of emotion in the clinical learning process, most of the focus of past research was on the ability of the supervisee to learn in a cognitive manner. For example, most clinical supervision models rely on the supervisee's ability to rationally think about a concept and apply it in the clinical environment.

Newer approaches to supervision likely will include multimodal forms of learning which include cognition and affective learning processes. How a clinician feels about a clinical situation will likely determine, at least partially, how he/she behaves in the situation. Further, experiencing negative emotions in a clinical situation has just as much impact, and maybe more, on the supervisee's learning as positive emotions.

Proposition Five

"Learning results from synergetic transactions between the person and the environment" (p. 194). Clinical learning occurs when a person interacts with their workplace environment. It is through the clinical act of assessment and treatment that disconnects occur and tacit beliefs are made explicit. It is the moment when the clinician realizes that his/her previous knowledge and experience are not sufficient to achieve the desired clinical outcome. The interplay between what one believes and what one experiences is learning in action. This interplay likely will emerge as the crux of learning through the supervisory process.

Proposition Six

"Learning is the process of creating knowledge" (p. 194). In the true constructivist paradigm, learning is the process of one's development of one's reality. Clinical learning occurs when the supervisee constructs her own reality based on individual clinical experiences and the thoughts, feelings, behaviors, and outcomes that occurred during those experiences. Taking a constructivist perspective toward clinical supervision leads the supervisor to focus on the supervisee's creation of her own knowledge base. This perspective, however, does not imply that an evidence base is absent in the supervisee's development of reality, truth, skill and knowledge. Instead, scholarly research is a strategy or resource the supervisee utilizes in the process of creating knowledge based on her clinical experiences.

Viewing clinical learning as a process of creating knowledge is in direct opposition to most clinical learning paradigms currently in use. The current approaches to supervision that view knowledge as something outside of the person, something the person strives to gather rather than to create, likely will be replaced with efforts to facilitate the development of the supervisee's ability to make sense of the clinical experience independently. Viewing knowledge as an external entity implies that knowledge is made up of perfectly understood facts that one must commit to memory. Instead, constructivist approaches to learning and knowing suggest that knowledge is created within the self and what traditionally is viewed as a fact is, in fact, subject to personal interpretation. Although such views may lead to ambiguity in clinical situations, ambiguity is what life is made of and what science is discovering to be the norm (Wheatley, 2006).

Measuring Supervisee Progress and Reactions to the Learning Process

Focusing on experiential learning processes rather than outcomes in clinical supervision brings to light one significant barrier to measuring supervisee development: *learning is an internal process that makes behavioral measurement challenging.* How the supervisor best and most efficiently measures and assesses the supervisee's progress in the learning process is an area rife for future research. Past research, however, may provide a good starting point. In fact, Jarvis (1987) developed a model of learning from experience which may prove useful in approaching clinical supervision from a process perspective. Jarvis described learning from experience as a set of nine potential responses to a learning situation. Of these nine potential responses, six are related to learning and three are related to nonlearning.

Nonlearning Responses

Presumption is a type of response one may give in which patterned behavior is elicited. According to Jarvis (1987), these patterned behaviors are a result of our socialization since birth and most people respond to social situations using these patterned responses. For example, in some cultures it is considered impolite to acknowledge a lack of understanding in a learning situation. If a student clinician from such a cultural background is unclear regarding what the supervisor is teaching in a clinical situation with a client, the student clinician may not seek further explanation during the clinical experience with the client (so as not to appear impolite). This response to a learning situation is a patterned response the student clinician learned through socialization.

Nonconsideration is another type of nonlearning response a supervisee may exhibit. Nonconsideration is synonymous with nonresponse, that is, the supervisee does not respond to a learning situation. There are many potential reasons why a supervisee may provide a non-response. Lack of time to consider the situation as well as concentrating on another matter rather than the present situation are just two possibilities.

Rejection of the learning situation is also a potential nonlearning response. Rejection of the learning situation is not the same response as nonconsideration. Instead, the supervisee rejects the potential to learn from a situation, despite having fully attended to it. For example, a clinician completing her clinical fellowship experience may believe that she can adequately assess a student's phonetic inventory through a non-structured story retell based on her previous experience with other children. Rather than attempting to test this belief with the current student to ascertain her ideas, she rejects the potential learning situation and carries on with the assessment after completion of the story retell without attempting to make sure the procedure met her assessment requirements. In measuring the clinician's response, whether or not the story retell was successful in adequately eliciting enough information to create a phonetic inventory is not as important as the clinician's rejection of the potential learning situation.

Nonreflective Learning Responses

Three of the six learning responses Jarvis described involve learning without reflection. Pre-conscious learning, practice, and memorization are all considered learning responses which lack an element of critical thought in learning. *Preconscious learning* occurs when no effort or conscious thought is put into learning from the situation. This type of learning is what Reber (1989) and Seger (1994) would term implicit learning. Responding to a clinical situation in which something new is learned without a conscious awareness of learning may be a difficult concept to grasp. Reber provided strong evidence for this type of learning through his experiments with the learning of artificial grammars. This type of learning response may take the form of a supervisee learning what to expect from their client's behavior without consciously or intentionally setting out to do so.

Practice is another of Jarvis' nonreflective learning responses. Practice is conscious but based on imitation. Often, supervisees may imitate a treatment approach based on their previous experiences observing other clinicians engage in the same or a similar approach to speech and language treatment. Although this form of learning is conscious and possibly useful, especially for the novice clinician, it is not a deeper form of learning. In fact, imitation lacks the critical stance a seasoned clinician would take when working with clients.

Last, *memorization* is a form of nonreflective learning. Although the uncritical addition of facts to one's memory is sometimes necessary (especially in traditional academic environments), memorization requires that a supervisee (and supervisor) accept that the "fact" is the only way one may view a concept. This type of learning is rarely useful in ambiguous, constantly changing clinical situations.

Reflective Learning Responses

Jarvis deemed the last three responses to a learning situation as a higher form of learning due to their reliance on more involved effort in the learning process. *Contemplation* is the process of thought. In fact, contemplation is a type of learning which Jarvis felt "the behaviorist definition omitted completely" (p. 33). Contemplation does not require a behavioral outcome; it is in and of itself the outcome.

Learning from a clinical situation through *reflective practice* is another response a supervisee may exhibit. Reflective practice is similar to a process of problem-solving. It involves conscious thought about the clinical situation, evaluation of possible solutions to a situation, and an assessment of the outcome of a particular clinical action. Reflective practice is synonymous with evidenced-based practice (Dollaghan, 2007) in speech-language pathology. This type of learning response is used to learn advanced skills and is elicited when there is a perceived gap in what a supervisee knows and what he/she feels is required in a clinical situation.

Last, *experimental learning* is based on humans' proclivity to constantly test their environments. This type of learning response serves to gain "knowledge that has been shown to relate to reality through experimentation" (p. 35). In the clinical supervisee, this type of response may be exhibited in two ways. First, the supervisee may test clinical hypotheses through this type of learning. Second, a supervisee may formally investigate theoretical hypotheses through experimental learning. Conducting research, at any level, is a form of experimental learning and is the crux of the evolving paradigm of the conduct of speech-language pathology through evidence-based practice.

Measuring supervisee progress, whether for a student or a new clinician, is necessary for a multitude of reasons. For the student, some type of progress evaluation is necessary to show the student's development over the semester and to assign a grade for the practicum experience. For the clinical fellow, it is necessary to show consistent development toward independent practice throughout the fellowship experience. Furthermore, the new or moderately experienced clinician also needs fair and consistent evaluation of clinical progress toward promotion within the organization. The supervisor dedicated to a process-based approach to supervision may use Jarvis' responses to the clinical learning situation as a means whereby the supervisee may be evaluated. Consistent reflective learning responses to new or challenging clinical situations is the benchmark for which the supervisee is striving.

However, it may be difficult to see the utility of such an approach at first glance. Most, if not all supervisors, have experienced the traditional, "supervisor as the wise party" approach to clinical supervision at this juncture in time. Such an approach assumes a finite body of knowledge ready to be shared with the supervisee. Realistically, however, clinical practice is made up of an infinite set of possibilities of client problems, personality traits, personal proclivities, work environments, changing patterns of accepted practice, and global health care or educational policy conditions. Ambiguity in the clinical process is the norm. The main goal of the supervisor is to facilitate the supervisee's ability to successfully navigate the myriad of possibilities the clinical situation is sure to provide.

In order to successfully prepare supervisees to deal with the challenge of ambiguous clinical situations, the supervisors would likely have been more successful if the supervisee's ability to learn in the workplace had been the focus of supervision from the start. However, there are often no "correct" answers in clinical work. Instead, the supervisee is required to navigate research, personal experience, and client wishes/values to make an educated decision that includes all three of these areas. A supervisee cannot be formally prepared for every single situation which may occur. Instead, through a focus on the clinical learning process, versus outcome, the supervisee becomes an independent decision maker adept at handling the unknown.

Final Thoughts: Evidence-Based Practice and the Future of Clinical Supervision

Although evidence-based practice as a driving force for clinical supervision was explored in earlier sections of this book, it is necessary to ascertain the current state of evidence-based practice and its potential to guide future directions in clinical supervision. The American Speech-Language-Hearing Association requires that speech-language pathologists (SLPs) incorporate evidence-based into their clinical activities (ASHA, 2004b, 2005). As Dollaghan (2007) and ASHA (2004b, 2005) described it, evidence-based practice makes use of evidence from external sources (research), clinical expertise, and patient/client values. Most research and writing regarding evidence-based practice, however, consists primarily of strategies in evaluating and using external evidence in clinical decision-making processes. Further difficulty in applying external evidence arises because research with highly specific subject selection criteria may possess reduced clinical applicability with diverse clinical populations (Elman, 2006). In cases where external evidence is based solely on homogeneous populations, the clinician would have to rely heavily, if not exclusively, on clinical expertise and patient/family values and beliefs.

However, research regarding how speech-language pathologists use clinical expertise and client/patient values and beliefs in clinical decision-making is almost nonexistent (save recent work by Skeat and Perry (2008) on clinicians' uses of outcomes measurement and

Hidecker, Jones, Imig, and Villarruel (2009) on using family paradigms to improve evidence-based practice). Referring to the dearth of research in the latter two areas of evidence-based practice is much more an observation than a critique. Rather, it is this author's hope that much more empirical effort will be directed toward the latter two sources of evidence in clinical decision-making.

Given the wealth of attention to external sources of data, in terms of evidence-based practice's role in clinical supervision, it is highly likely that most principles of evidence-based practice that are infused into clinical supervision are based on the evaluation and use of external evidence. Therefore, effective evaluation and use of both internal (clinical experience) and patient/caregiver sources of data are likely neglected—the research to guide clinical supervision in these latter two areas of evidence-based practice simply does not exist. In fact, Worrall and Bennett (2001) found that clinicians perceive incongruence between external evidence and clinical realities. Allmark (1995) described just such sentiments as the *theory-practice gap*. According to Allmark (1995), a theory-practice gap occurs when attempts are made to describe practice as applied theory. He refers to the Greek origins of both theory and practice and points out that the Ancient Greeks had different terms for the types of knowledge included in theory and practice. In Allmark's (1995) classical view, theory informs practice; however, practice in and of itself requires other types of knowledge. Jarvis (2000), himself, found that teaching theory that can be directly applied to a clinical situation presupposes that practice situations do not change. It is clear that practice situations, however, do change—if not constantly.

So what can the clinical supervisor do to facilitate supervisees' successful negotiation of ever changing clinical situations and environments while instilling the values and practices of evidence-based practice? Use of strategies that incorporate the historical with the future likely will facilitate holistic growth in supervisees— the type of growth that allows more independent learning in the workplace. Clinical supervision strategies that facilitate such growth include cognitive learning principles, affective learning considerations, and a focus on experiential learning. The concepts outlined in this chapter one hopes, will serve to spark interest in the use of theory in experiential learning as well as integration of traditional approaches to supervision with broader, more encompassing perspectives on the clinical learning process.

This chapter takes a unique perspective in that it considers the role of the adult learner in the process of supervision and mentorship. The adult learner comes to the clinical training situation with life experiences and questions that other learners lack. They want to know why they are learning a particular concept and how it applies to prior knowledge. They are in a sense "re-learning" each time they learn in a process of continual comparing new information with their own unique set of experiences. It is important for clinical educators to take into account the learning styles of their clinicians to achieve the best benefit and satisfaction for all. In this fashion, using the data regarding adult learners enhances a systematic approach to supervision and mentorship.

What's Next?

In the following chapter, the reader is guided through a summation and concluding thoughts regarding supervision and mentorship.

Reflective Assignment

At this point, readers are encouraged to begin developing a database of their own personal supervision experiences. This may include good experiences as well as struggles and challenges. Reflect on each of the situations and how they were handled. You may use the space below to begin jotting down your thoughts:

_____

_____

_____

_____

_____

_____

_____

_____

_____

_____

_____

_____

_____

_____

_____

_____

_____

_____

_____

_____

_____

CHAPTER 11

Conclusions

We make a living by what we get, we make a life by what we give.

Winston Churchill

The purpose of this chapter is to conclude and review some of the salient points raised in the preceding chapters regarding the importance of recognizing and analyzing the scientific underpinnings of the study of research. The chapters have examined historical framework, leading scholarship, competencies and skills, and various underlying issues impacting supervision and mentorship in increasingly complex clinical domains.

Competency-based supervision practice draws from many sources both from within the speech-language pathology and externally. This is a notion with national as well as international roots (Ferguson, 2008). Communication specialists draw on research about the process of communication in terms of linguistic dyads to observe, analyze, and improve the specific of instructional dialogue in the clinical supervision setting. This is in addition to the vast array of literature accumulating in this area via ASHA and independent research. Is there a science to successful supervision and mentorship? The answer is "yes."

In short, there has been a great deal of scientific evidence gathered regarding the activities that make up supervision. The research extends back over several decades, and in many ways, current thinking continues to reflect many of the sound foundational tenets of our organization. This information forms the foundation of a pedagogically focused approach to supervision and seeks to combine research with clinical experience in a systematic way, in keeping with our training on research synthesis on any topic in our purview.

The ASHA guidelines for certification (2010b), as well as individual licensure standards, are the standards to which all speech-language pathology professionals must adhere. It is the area of interpretation both in student level and throughout the career span that this book hopes to shed light on.

As supervision is an area of study onto itself, SLP professionals must follow the same steps to define a problem, gather relevant evidence, and determine the specific clinical aspects that can lead to sound decision-making in any supervisory situation. Care to practice supervision in a systematic fashion is essential in the growth of the supervisor, the supervisee, and ultimately the benefit of our clients, which is of primary concern.

The works cited in this book cover a chronology of the scientific explorations and explanations of the components of supervision. Recognizing the interpersonal dynamics involved in clinical supervision, the comparison of teaching models in terms of group versus one-to-one supervision was examined by Dowling (1983, 1987). This observation of supervisory outcomes was very important in that it recognized a critical component, "self-supervisory talk" behavior. As the goal of supervision is to work toward a model of relative independence, this early study was very valuable in its research goal.

This is in keeping with the work reported by Shapiro and Anderson (1989), who reported that supervision consists of a set of structured activities introduced early in the young clinical career and then gradually faded to the point of self-supervision and reflection. The methodologies of supervision have been examined and continue to be major points of research. As an example, Zanello, in her 1989 dissertation, compared outcomes of students who were supervised with videotape playback versus those with whom direct observation was used. She cites the use of formats such as questionnaires and feedback forms developed by earlier researchers as manner by which to gain and compare data.

Gillam, Roussos, and Anderson (1990) described many similar evaluative elements that serve to objectify exactly what it means to supervise and which factors can be identified as quality indicators. Gillam and colleagues (1990) drew on a great deal of past research, notably Glaser and Donnelly (1989), who discussed the need for training to be an effective self-supervisor in speech pathology. Another earlier work which influenced the current study was conducted by Goldhammer as early as 1969 (and Cogan in 1973), which describes educational supervision models in general. Gillam and colleagues (1990) stated that target behaviors improve after they become the focus of supervision. This indicates that the outcome of supervision may be studied and tracked, just as our behavioral outcomes for students, increasing evidence-based components to our practice.

Many resources that were available to the study of supervision continue in much more highly developed forums. Of particular interest is the journal published by Routledge Press, *The Clinical Supervisor*, which presents research components of supervision from an interdisciplinary perspective. For ASHA members such as myself, we benefit from many avenues, in particular the activities of Special Interest Division 11 which provides leadership to professionals interested in SLP supervision.

In an effort to provide a current review of research in this area, the following authors are cited, although this area is one of ongoing research. Many call for continued efforts in various arenas of research. However, systematic review of levels of evidence is difficult to accomplish in that the nature of research questions asked, and the methodology used, vary so considerably. However, within-study analysis indicates a strong level of outcome support due to rigor in which our discipline writes and publishes.

Within the last decade, in particular, there has been a significant amount of research published. Back in 2002, Pershey studied how client feedback regarding effectiveness can assist in the training of clinicians as well as their supervisors. This provides a key variable as an indicator for individual indices that a center or clinic can include in a self-study.

A comprehensive article by Wren Newman, Coordinator of ASHA's Administration and Supervision Division 11, titled, "The Basics of Supervision," (2005) is a foundational reading for speech-language pathologists and audiologists as it provides a clear stage by stage analysis of the chief tasks of supervision and ethical components, as well as teaching cases.

It is of interest to note that Zipoli, in the same year (2005), reported that clinical experience as well as opinions of other practitioners are used more frequently to guide clinical decision-making rather than research studies in supervision and clinical practice guidelines. There is less reliance on evidence-based practice notions once clinicians graduate, and the merging of evidence bases and clinical experience is a task that supervisors must train and a skill to develop. It may be that the clinicians do not have time/energy resources to delve into comprehensive reviews of literature. However, if the profession is to be grounded in science, we must adhere to the principles that treatment designs tested in larger populations with greater controls will contribute to our supervisory expertise. It is important that a new and ongoing supervisor be familiar with the controversies and dilemmas in supervision, separate and apart from his or her own technical knowledge of a given population, particularly in training institutions.

In 2006, two additional papers appeared that shed continued light on the critical subject of availability of student training situations in general (Johnson, 2006) as well as the dissertation by Clemente (2006) that discussed how clinicians can improve in self-sufficiency. Grounded in the Jean Anderson model of supervision, Clemente (2006) found that self-sufficiency is increased if supervisors use consultative as opposed to teacher or counselor roles. Very important, however, is the fact that the supervisory style must evolve and be suited to the level of student training. As in all studies of supervision, the individual variables of the student background and prior exposure to training is critical, and individual.

Goldstein (2008) and Gillam and Gillam (2008) all speak to notion of the quantification and qualification of supervision. Goldstein reported that evidence-based practice training of students involves the supervisors helping students connect with the research and attempt to classify research to apply it more effectively. This can be constructed both at a training level as well as in early practice and eventually as a self-driven vehicle to "best practice." Gillam and Gillam (2008) further describe the major steps to applying evidence-based practice that can help guide supervisory intervention. These include: learning how to ask the central clinical question, locating research and evaluating research evidence, as well as identifying and integrating individual clinical experience and client related factors.

Research presented by O'Connor (2008) reinforces these notions as she states that supervision evolves and the amount and type of supervision will grow and change with good practice. Ostergren, in a 2008 dissertation, continues that supervision is generally studied in a student context. A supervisor, however, may become a mentor. Self-awareness on the part of the supervisor may grow using models from other disciplines such as counseling. In addition, indicators of achievement, such as supervisory styles, may encompass inventories drawn from earlier work by Friedlander, discussed in Ward (1984). Essentially, it is the task of the supervisor and the student or clinician to simultaneously integrate data from multiple sources in a systematic fashion that contributes to good clinical decision-making by all parties. Teaching students how to integrate data (Epstein, 2008) and to be sensitive to these principles can be very fundamental to effective supervision and independence. Throughout this book, information such as reflective practice, conversational styles, data collection and the concern for level and background of the student or clinician are discussed in terms of how this may be accomplished.

A recent study conducted by Ho and Whitehill (2009) reported on a way to increase the effectiveness of supervision and found that immediate verbal feedback increased effectiveness of supervision. By applying this and above practices, the astute young supervisor can utilize the results of supervisory research that has been studied and put to scientific test.

In addition to published research, supervision has also been the subject of current dissertation research. A recent example comes out of Nova Southeastern University, which has produced several doctoral dissertations pertaining to clinical supervision. A study conducted by Carol Koch (2009), entitled, "A Qualitative Investigation Examining the Effect of Supervisory Feedback on the Development of Clinicians' Expertise," analyzed aspects such as the amount of content information and technical information in the supervisory comments.

Ferguson (2010) writes about the "pivotal moment" in clinical work and the critical importance of using all resources, particularly in the act of appraisal, necessary in supervision, and the importance of communication and interaction that can be studied linguistically to enhance supervision.

The central question of this book is to investigate the ways in which supervision and mentorship in speech pathology can be objectified for purposes of effective training paradigms. This question has had many answers and approaches spanning several decades as the profession grew. Oratio (1977) wrote on this topic and many of his thoughts are very similar to current writings. He included case studies, examples of supervisory dialogues and offered insights into the self-reflective process.

In contrast, the much more current book edited by Roddam and Skeat (2010) contains an in-depth synthesis of evidence based approaches to many areas of speech pathology practice, including a chapter about supervision by Hannah Crawford (2007) who described a model of evidence-based practice. Crawford (2007) presents case supervision scenarios that incorporate the components of evidence-based practice; namely, patient preference, clinical experience, and best available evidence. These principles can be utilized to determine optimal clinical decision-making and demonstrate that models of supervision can be driven by objective methodologies.

In the goal of establishing the science behind supervision, the American Speech-Language and Hearing Association has reported that evidence-based knowledge about practice in clinical supervision has come primarily from descriptive studies (ASHA, 2004b). These reports have led to knowledge about behaviors that appear to facilitate supervision and growth of supervisees in problem-solving. The report also indicates that much information has been gleaned from other disciplines and contributed to acknowledgment of shared principles (ASHA, 2008a).

Importantly, ASHA in the same document provides a current definition of supervision that draws on earlier models but is extended to include development of intrapersonal skills such as self-analysis and self-evaluation. Additionally, the critical aspect of intercultural factors are emphasized in order to achieve the best social dynamic in the supervision process. The resources provided by Gunther (n.d.) provide a wealth of information on the whole range of issues surrounding supervision for individuals at all stages of their career.

Data collection in supervision may be accomplished through a variety of measures, and can be individually designed. In the clinical fellowship year, the document known as the Clinical Fellowship Skills Inventory developed by ASHA is used to document abilities in evaluation, therapy, and management areas. The practice of supervision is enhanced when the supervisor has had work and educational experience in how to supervise. Expanded offerings in the area of clinical supervision are provided as continuing education and conference proceedings so that new and continuing supervisors can improve their practice.

According to ASHA, the mentoring component of supervision may be most appropriate in later-stage supervision when the student/clinician has moved towards self-supervision for basic service delivery and is facing more challenging professional issues. The supervisory-mentorship continuum is well described by Melanie Hudson, (2009) in her presentations to the Pennsylvania and Florida state speech associations. The shared principles of supervision and mentorship, the importance of collaborative teaching models and the goals of self-evaluation for both partners are emphasized in her work.

The scrutiny of evidence-based practice has been applied to supervision studies as shown by the work of Lee-Wilkerson and Chabon [ASHA's incoming president], (2008) who reported on a rubric to facilitate accurate student reflective practice. This notion was reinforced by the work of Mary Pat McCarthy (2009, 2010) who reported that performance indicators and written reflections were successful in enhancing graduate students' reflective practice. Independent practice is enhanced via the available of technical resources via the Internet. Clinicians can update their education very readily in all areas of practice. There also is an increase in evidence-based practice journals such as the EBP Briefs published by Pearson that refers to clinical areas (see Justice & Pence, 2007 for an example). The ability to synthesize all the material may be enhanced by methodologies such as software for comparing research.

In reviewing this body of research, it may be concluded that there are many factors to define during the complex processes of supervision and mentorship, and no one approach can be recommended without individual modifications. Just as in clinical practice, the study of supervision and mentorship necessarily involves the gathering of data and the comparison of research findings. A parallel exists between the steps in a clinical practice whether you are a clinician or a supervisor. We ask the critical questions about the situation, acquire the best evidence, and appraise it for applicability. We then apply the evidence in the context of our clinical setting, including our client preferences, and assess the outcome and share it with our professional community.

Despite all of the challenges and complexities of this process as have been described throughout this book, the growth of a relationship from supervisor to mentor can be one of the most rewarding in our profession. It is hoped that the resources contained herein and insights from the many contributions will advance the science of supervision.

This book has attempted to elucidate certain learning principles that a new student or clinician can expect to experience with their supervisor. Similarly, the new or returning supervisor can draw on the information provided in this book. It is up to the colleagues who read and respond to the themes of this book to extract from it what is new or reaffirming. This will further contribute to the goals of best supervision, best care, and best careers for all of us. There is a growing body of evidence from research that supports how modern supervision can be both productive and satisfying, as well as grounded in knowledge and evidence-based practice.

The author of this book hopes that she may have succeeded in the goal of shedding light on a multifaceted challenge in the clinical field of speech-language pathology delivery of services and supervision. There is no one solution. However, by compiling collective information, we can examine the short- and long-term responses so that future clinicians, supervisors, and mentors may take initiative to seek depth and breadth solutions in the work-place. It is a starting point that I hope stimulates ongoing dialogue regarding reflective practice in supervision and mentorship in our beloved profession.

Reflective Assignment

Based on everything you have read thus far, it is my hope that you will take all of the information and ideas presented in this book and use them in guiding your own thinking and practice. At this point, readers are encouraged to begin writing a personal/professional time line as a means of reflecting on one's own experiences, both past and present. Readers are also encouraged to generate several personal/professional goals for the future, as a means of further enhancing growth and development as a mentor and supervisor. Please use the space provided below:

FUTURE GOALS

1.
2.
3.
4.
5.
6.

APPENDIXES

In this section, readers will find several examples of rating scales and evaluation instruments that can be very useful to implement during supervision. These may be used as a means to formally assess performance and/or as an informal evaluation tool. The questions and issues raised in these instruments offer supervisors the opportunity to engage students in reflective thinking and self-analysis, which is one of the main end goals of successful supervision, as discussed throughout this book. These instruments also may be helpful to use as a platform from which to base a dialogue regarding the overall supervisory process and clinical experience. The ASHA Knowledge and Skills document as well as the Clinical Fellowship Skills Inventory are also provided as they list important skill areas and competencies that a supervisee is expected to master at the completion of their clinical experience. It is hoped that readers will find these instruments helpful and will make use of them in their own clinical practice.

APPENDIX A

Division 11 Supervisor Credential Survey Results

Additional Analyses by Selected Primary
Employment Facility Categories

1. What is your experience in supervision? (Check all that apply.)

	All respondents (n=406)		School (n=46)		College/ university (n=189)		Hospital (n=71)		Non-residential HC (n=49)	
	%	#	%	#	%	#	%	#	%	#
None	0.5%	2	—	0	—	0	—	0	2.0%	1
Graduate students	88.9%	361	67.4%	31	97.9%	185	87.3%	62	85.7%	42
Clinical Fellows	68.7%	279	82.6%	38	62.4%	118	76.1%	54	69.4%	34
Audiology/speech-language pathology practitioners	55.2%	224	56.5%	26	43.4%	82	80.3%	57	55.1%	27
Paraprofessionals/ assistants/aides	35.0%	142	60.9%	28	19.6%	37	39.4%	28	49.0%	24
Other professionals	25.6%	104	—	—	—	—	—	—	—	—

2. What kind of training have you received in supervision? (Check all that apply.)

	All respondents (n=406)		School (n=46)		College/ university (n=189)		Hospital (n=71)		Non-residential HC (n=49)	
	%	#	%	#	%	#	%	#	%	#
None	1.5%	6	—	0	2.1%	4	2.8%	2	—	0
Informal networking	65.0%	264	54.3%	25	68.8%	130	62.0%	44	63.3%	31
Self study/readings	85.0%	345	80.4%	37	88.4%	167	85.9%	61	79.6%	39
Workshops/conferences	75.6%	307	60.9%	28	82.5%	156	71.8%	51	67.3%	33
On-the-job training	76.8%	312	71.7%	33	76.2%	144	80.3%	57	69.4%	34
College or university courses for credit	18.7%	76	32.6%	15	16.4%	31	16.9%	12	12.2%	6
Other	9.6%	39	—	—	—	—	—	—	—	—

3. How important is formal training in supervision?

	All respondents (n=404)		School (n=46)		College/ university (n=189)		Hospital (n=71)		Non-residential HC (n=49)	
	%	#	%	#	%	#	%	#	%	#
Very important	67.6%	273	67.4%	31	70.9%	134	60.6%	43	65.3%	32
Somewhat important	29.5%	119	28.3%	13	26.5%	50	35.2%	25	34.7%	17
Minimally important	2.0%	8	2.2%	1	2.1%	4	1.4%	1	—	0
Not at all important	0.2%	1	—	0	—	0	1.4%	1	—	0
Do not know/no opinion	0.7%	3	2.2%	1	0.5%	1	1.4%	1	—	0

4. Who would benefit from formal training in supervision? (Check all that apply.)

	All respondents (n=404)		School (n=46)		College/ university (n=189)		Hospital (n=71)		Non-residential HC (n=49)	
	%	#	%	#	%	#	%	#	%	#
New supervisors	98.3%	397	95.7%	44	98.9%	187	100%	71	93.9%	46
Current supervisors with no formal training	93.1%	376	91.3%	42	93.7%	177	91.5%	65	89.8%	44
Current supervisors interested in additional training	97.0%	392	97.8%	45	96.8%	183	97.2%	69	98.0%	48
Experienced supervisors	74.8%	302	71.7%	33	78.3%	148	74.6%	53	63.3%	31
Other	7.2%	29	—		—		—		—	

5. What kind of training in supervision would you participate in, if available? (Check all that apply.)

	All respondents (*n* = 404)		School (*n* = 46)		College/ university (*n* = 189)		Hospital (*n* = 71)		Non-residential HC (*n* = 49)	
	%	#	%	#	%	#	%	#	%	#
None	1.0%	4	2.2%	1	0.5%	1	—	0	2.0%	1
Self study/readings	83.9%	339	80.4%	37	84.1%	159	84.5%	60	83.7%	41
Workshops/conferences	96.0%	388	95.7%	44	98.4%	186	94.4%	67	93.9%	46
College or university courses for credit	40.1%	162	47.8%	22	43.9%	83	28.2%	20	32.7%	16
Other	11.9%	48	—	—	—	—	—	—	—	—

6. If a course of study existed in the area of supervision leading to a credential, how likely is it that you would participate?

	All respondents (*n* = 403)		School (*n* = 46)		College/ university (*n* = 189)		Hospital (*n* = 71)		Non-residential HC (*n* = 49)	
	%	#	%	#	%	#	%	#	%	#
Very likely	53.3%	215	56.5%	26	55.6%	105	46.5%	33	46.9%	23
More likely than unlikely	33.7%	136	32.6%	15	31.2%	59	38.0%	27	42.9%	21
More unlikely than likely	4.5%	18	2.2%	1	6.3%	12	1.4%	1	4.1%	2
Very unlikely	5.5%	22	4.3%	2	4.8%	9	8.5%	6	6.1%	3
Do not know/no opinion	3.0%	12	4.3%	2	2.1%	4	5.6%	4	—	0

7. What factors would influence your decision to pursue a credential in supervision? (Check all that apply.)

	All respondents (n=402)		School (n=46)		College/ university (n=189)		Hospital (n=71)		Non-residential HC (n=49)	
	%	#	%	#	%	#	%	#	%	#
Amount of time required	82.6%	332	67.4%	31	82.5%	156	90.1%	64	77.6%	38
Cost	83.1%	334	84.8%	39	84.7%	160	87.3%	62	67.3%	33
Enhanced career opportunities	37.3%	150	56.5%	26	27.5%	52	35.2%	25	44.9%	22
Increased knowledge and skills in supervision	75.9%	305	76.1%	35	72.5%	137	74.6%	53	87.8%	43
Professional commitment	47.8%	192	54.3%	25	50.3%	95	39.4%	28	42.9%	21
Recognition of credential by employer(s)	48.0%	193	52.2%	24	47.6%	90	47.9%	34	38.8%	19
Travel (if required)	51.2%	206	47.8%	22	48.7%	92	57.7%	41	51.0%	25
Other	7.5%	30	—	—	—	—	—	—	—	—

8. What format would you consider for training leading to a credential in supervision? (Check all that apply.)

	All respondents (n = 400)		School (n = 46)		College/ university (n = 189)		Hospital (n = 71)		Non-residential HC (n = 49)	
	%	#	%	#	%	#	%	#	%	#
Online professional development	85.3%	341	89.1%	41	84.7%	160	78.9%	56	85.7%	42
Face-to-face professional development workshop	78.0%	312	76.1%	35	76.2%	144	73.2%	52	81.6%	40
Face-to-face session(s)/ short course in conjunction with face-to-face national convention/ conferences	62.0%	248	41.3%	19	69.3%	131	56.3%	40	59.2%	29
Session(s)/short course in conjunction with state conventions	70.0%	280	67.4%	31	75.1%	142	63.4%	45	65.3%	32
Other	7.3%	29	—	—	—	—	—	—	—	—

9. What is the maximum number of hours that you would be willing to spend in coursework or other instructional activities that lead to a credential in supervision?

	All respondents (n = 383)	School (n = 46)	College/ university (n = 189)	Hospital (n = 71)	Non- residential HC (n = 49)
Mean	25.5	22.0	25.7	26.2	22.0
Median	20.0	20.0	20.0	24.0	20.0
Standard deviation	27.1	17.6	28.6	26.6	21.4
Range	0–200	2–100	0–200	0–200	0–100

10. What is your professional area? (Check all that apply.)

	All respondents (n = 403)		School (n = 46)		College/ university (n = 189)		Hospital (n = 71)		Non-residential HC (n = 49)	
	%	#	%	#	%	#	%	#	%	#
Audiology	5.5%	22	—	0	7.9%	15	5.6%	4	4.1%	2
Speech-language pathology	94.3%	380	97.8%	45	93.7%	177	93.0%	66	91.8%	45
Speech/language/hearing science	2.7%	11	2.2%	1	1.1%	2	5.6%	4	8.2%	4
Other	2.7%	11	6.6%	3	1.0%	2	2.8%	2	4.0%	2

Victor, S. (2010). Coordinator's column. Perspectives on *Administration and Supervision, 20*(3), 83–84.

APPENDIX B

Clinical Fellowship Skills Inventory (CFSI)

Speech-Language Pathology

Description Of The Inventory

The CFSI consists of 18 skill statements covering four areas: (a) evaluation, (b) treatment, (c) management, and (d) interaction. The rating scale for each skill has been designed along a 5-point continuum, ranging from "5" (representing the most effective performance) to "1" (representing the least effective performance). Approval of the clinical fellowship requires a minimum rating of "3" on the core skills during the last segment in which the core skill is rated. **Core skills are noted on the inventory with an asterisk** (*). The clinical fellowship supervisor will match the clinical fellow's performance to the descriptor for each skill. The rating for one skill need not be the same as the ratings for other skills. For each skill included on the CFSI the CF supervisor will decide which point on the scale best reflects the performance of the clinical fellow during the segment being rated. (Because the clinical fellowship is divided into three equal segments, each segment represents one third of the total experience.) **The fellowship supervisor must complete the inventory at least once during each of the three segments of the clinical fellowship.** The category "Not Applicable (NA)" appears on two items of the rating scale and may be used only for these items. **NA should be used only if the facility does not provide an opportunity for the fellow to perform the**

skill during the segment. However, the CF supervisor is encouraged to coordinate the observation schedule to ensure that all applicable skills are observed and evaluated.

Rating Tips

To determine the rating for **each** skill, consider the fellow's effectiveness in working with specific client populations in terms of client's (a) age (infants, children, adults), (b) type and severity of communication disorder, (c) physical limitations, (d) cultural background, (e) English proficiency, (f) literacy level, and (g) alternative communication system use. In addition to considering these factors for all skills, Skill 4 and Skill 10 have been included to evaluate the clinical fellow's ability to **adapt** all testing and treatment procedures on the basis of these factors. To distinguish among the fellow's performance levels (from 5, representing most effective performance, to 1, representing least effective performance), read the descriptors carefully and consider the following four factors, when applicable, in relation to the skill being rated:

Accuracy—the degree to which the clinical fellow performs a skill without error

Consistency—the degree to which the clinical fellow performs a skill at the same level of proficiency across cases

Independence—the degree to which the clinical fellow performs a skill in a self-directed manner

Supervisory Guidance—the degree to which the clinical fellow seeks consultations when needed.

Rating accuracy depends on the frequency, duration, and range of the fellowship supervisor's observations of the fellow's performance. One of the most important factors associated with rating accuracy is the opportunity to observe relevant behaviors. Rating accuracy will be greatest when the supervisor and the fellow interact frequently on the job and the fellowship supervisor has many opportunities to observe critical work behaviors. Rating accuracy also depends on the familiarity of the fellowship supervisor and the fellow with the Clinical Fellowship Skills Inventory. The fellowship supervisor must observe the on-the-job performance of the fellow, and both supervisor and fellow must understand the rating process and procedures described in the Handbook. Choose the one descriptor that best describes the clinical fellow's performance and circle the corresponding number on the Clinical Fellowship Report form. Options are available (ratings 4 and 2) for describing performance that falls between two adjacent descriptors.

Do not submit the following form. Use the Clinical Fellowship Report and Rating Form (Form D) to record fellows' rating on each skill.

Evaluation Skills

1. Implements screening procedures.

RATING	DESCRIPTOR
☐ 5	CF independently and accurately matches and/or adapts screening procedures to all populations, selects appropriate screening criteria, administers and scores screening instrument(s) efficiently, interprets results, and makes appropriate recommendations. CF seeks supervisory guidance if needed.
☐ 4	
☐ 3	CF independently and accurately matches and/or adapts screening procedures to most populations, selects appropriate screening criteria, administers and scores screening instrument(s), interprets results, and makes appropriate recommendations. CF usually seeks supervisory guidance when needed.

RATING	DESCRIPTOR
☐ 2	
☐ 1	CF requires supervisory guidance to accurately match and/or adapt screening procedures to populations and to select appropriate screening criteria. CF may demonstrate difficulty in administering and scoring screening instrument(s), and/or interpreting results, and making appropriate recommendations. CF does not seek supervisory guidance when needed.

*2. **Collects case history information and integrates information from client, family, caregivers, significant others, and professionals.**

RATING	DESCRIPTOR
☐ 5	CF independently and accurately selects case history or other interview formats with consideration for all relevant factors. CF efficiently collects and spontaneously probes for additional relevant information, obtains information from other sources, and integrates data in order to identify etiologic and/or contributing factors. CF seeks supervisory guidance if needed.
☐ 4	
☐ 3	In most situations, CF independently and accurately selects case history or other interview formats with consideration for all relevant factors. CF collects and probes for additional information, obtains information from other sources, and integrates data to identify etiologic and/or contributing factors. CF usually seeks supervisory guidance when needed.
☐ 2	

RATING	DESCRIPTOR
☐ 1	CF requires supervisory guidance to accurately select case history or other interview formats with consideration for all relevant factors. CF collects case history information that is incomplete or lacking in relevance. CF is unable to integrate data to identify etiologic and/or other contributing factors and does not seek supervisory guidance when needed.

*3. Selects and implements evaluation procedures (nonstandardized tests, behavioral observations, and standardized tests).

RATING	DESCRIPTOR
☐ 5	CF independently selects a comprehensive assessment battery with consideration for all relevant factors. CF efficiently and accurately administers the battery and consistently scores tests accurately. CF seeks supervisory guidance if needed.
☐ 4	
☐ 3	In most situations, CF independently selects an adequate assessment battery (i.e., basic procedures needed to define problem adequately) with consideration for all relevant factors. CF administers the battery, scores tests accurately, and usually seeks supervisory guidance when needed.
☐ 2	
☐ 1	CF requires supervisory guidance to select evaluation procedures that are appropriate and complete. CF may administer and/or score tests inaccurately and does not seek supervisory guidance when needed.

*4. Adapts interviewing and testing procedures to meet individual client needs.

RATING	DESCRIPTOR
☐ 5	CF independently and accurately recognizes when testing procedures need to be adapted to accommodate needs unique to specific clients. Effectively implements appropriate adaptations, and makes maximum use of all available resources to provide for unusual situations. CF seeks supervisory guidance if needed.
☐ 4	
☐ 3	In most situations CF independently and accurately recognizes when testing procedures need to be adapted to accommodate needs unique to specific clients and implements appropriate modifications. May need assistance in accessing available resources. CF usually seeks supervisory guidance when needed.
☐ 2	
☐ 1	CF requires supervisory guidance to recognize the need for and/or to adapt procedures to accommodate individual needs. CF does not seek supervisory guidance when needed.

*5. Interprets and integrates test results and behavioral observations, synthesizes information gained from all sources, develops diagnostic impressions, and makes recommendations.

RATING	DESCRIPTOR
☐ 5	CF consistently, independently, and accurately interprets and integrates test results and behavioral observations to define the client's communicative functioning, which includes relating etiologic factors to observed behaviors and test results. CF consistently develops diagnostic impressions and makes comprehensive recommendations leading to appropriate case management. CF seeks supervisor guidance if needed.
☐ 4	
☐ 3	In most situations, CF independently and accurately interprets and integrates test results and behavioral observations to define the client's communicative functioning. CF develops diagnostic impressions and makes basic recommendations that are consistent with evaluation results and that are adequate for case management. CF usually seeks supervisory guidance when needed.
☐ 2	
☐ 1	CF requires supervisory guidance to interpret diagnostic data and/or behavioral observations accurately. Diagnostic impressions and/or recommendations are either absent, inappropriate, or inconsistent with evaluation results. CF does not seek supervisory guidance when needed.

Treatment Skills

6. Develops and implements specific, reasonable, and necessary treatment plans.

RATING	DESCRIPTOR
☐ 5	CF independently and accurately establishes a treatment plan appropriate for the client. CF consistently develops specific and reasonable treatment plans that include long-term goals and measurable short-term objectives which reflect appropriate learning sequence, identifies the most appropriate settings for service, explores all alternative service delivery options, and effectively implements plans. CF seeks supervisory guidance if needed.
☐ 4	
☐ 3	In most situations, CF independently and accurately establishes treatment plans appropriate for the client. The treatment plan includes long-term goals and measurable short-term objectives, which usually reflect a logical sequencing of learning steps. CF generally identifies the need to explore alternative service delivery options, but may need help in selecting the most appropriate options. CF can effectively implement planned procedures. CF usually seeks supervisory guidance when needed.
☐ 2	

RATING	DESCRIPTOR
☐ 1	CF requires supervisory guidance to accurately develop a treatment plan appropriate for the client. The treatment plan may include adequate long-term goals, but objectives are not measurable and/or do not reflect logical sequencing of learning steps. CF cannot identify appropriate service delivery options and, even with guidance, may not effectively implement treatment plans. CF does not seek supervisory guidance when needed.

7. Selects/develops and implements intervention strategies for treatment of communication and related disorders.

RATING	DESCRIPTOR
☐ 5	CF independently and consistently selects/develops materials and instrumentation for which there is a clear rationale and uses these materials and instrumentation creatively and effectively to enhance the treatment process. CF seeks supervisory guidance if needed.
☐ 4	
☐ 3	In most situations, CF independently selects/develops and implements intervention strategies relevant to the communication disorder and the unique characteristics of the client. CF usually seeks supervisory guidance when needed.
☐ 2	
☐ 1	CF requires supervisory guidance to select/develop and/or implement intervention strategies relevant to the needs of the client. CF does not seek supervisory guidance when needed.

*8. **Selects/develops and uses intervention materials and instrumentation for treatment of communication and related disorders.**

RATING	DESCRIPTOR
☐ 5	CF independently and consistently selects/develops materials and instrumentation for which there is a clear rationale and uses these materials and instrumentation creatively and effectively to enhance the treatment process. CF seeks supervisory guidance if needed.
☐ 4	
☐ 3	In most situations, CF independently selects/develops materials and instrumentation that are relevant to the communication disorder and uses materials and/or instrumentation effectively. CF usually seeks supervisory guidance when needed.
☐ 2	
☐ 1	CF requires supervisory guidance to select materials and/or instrumentation that are appropriate to the treatment objectives, client, and/or the activity. Once selected, CF may not use materials and/or instrumentation effectively. CF does not seek supervisory guidance when needed.

*9. **Plans and implements a program of periodic monitoring of the client's communicative functioning through the use of appropriate data collection systems. Interprets and uses data to modify treatment plans, strategies, materials, and/or instrumentation to meet the needs of the client.**

RATING	DESCRIPTOR
☐ 5	CF independently develops and implements a comprehensive program of periodic monitoring of the client's communicative functioning and collects and interprets data accurately. Uses this information to effectively modify treatment plans, strategies, materials, and/or instrumentation to meet the needs of the client. CF seeks supervisory guidance if needed.
☐ 4	
☐ 3	In most situations, CF independently develops and implements a program of periodic monitoring of the client's communicative functioning. Collects and interprets data accurately and uses this information to modify treatment plans, strategies, materials, and/or instrumentation to meet the needs of the client. CF usually seeks supervisory guidance when needed.
☐ 2	
☐ 1	CF requires supervisory guidance to plan and implement a program of periodic monitoring of the client's communicative functioning. CF does not collect useful and/or accurate data in order to modify treatment plans, strategies, materials, and/or instrumentation to meet the needs of the client. CF does not seek supervisory guidance when needed.

*10. **Adapts intervention procedures, strategies, materials, and instrumentation to meet individual client needs.**

RATING	DESCRIPTOR
☐ 5	CF independently and consistently adapts intervention procedures, strategies, materials, and instrumentation to accommodate needs unique to specific clients. Makes maximum use of all available resources to provide for unusual situations. CF effectively implements appropriate adaptations and seeks supervisory guidance if needed.
☐ 4	
☐ 3	CF recognizes when intervention procedures, strategies, materials, and/or instrumentation need to be adapted to accommodate needs unique to specific clients. May need assistance in making appropriate adaptations. CF usually seeks supervisory guidance when needed.
☐ 2	
☐ 1	CF requires supervisory guidance to recognize the need for adaptation of intervention procedures, strategies, materials, and/or instrumentation to accommodate needs unique to specific clients. CF may have difficulty implementing identified adaptations and does not seek supervisory guidance when needed.

Management Skills

*11. Schedules and prioritizes direct and indirect service activities, maintains client records, and documents professional contacts and clinical reports in a timely manner.

RATING	DESCRIPTOR
☐ 5	CF independently and consistently prioritizes activities, schedules client contacts and meetings, maintains client records accurately, and makes and documents professional contacts in a timely manner. CF seeks supervisory guidance if needed.
☐ 4	
☐ 3	CF independently prioritizes most activities, consistently schedules client contacts and meetings, maintains client records accurately, and usually makes and documents professional contacts in a timely manner. CF usually seeks supervisory guidance when needed.
☐ 2	
☐ 1	CF requires supervisory guidance to prioritize activities, schedule client contacts and meetings, maintain client records, and make professional contacts in a timely manner. CF does not seek supervisory guidance when needed.

12. **Complies with program administrative and other regulatory policies such as required due process documentation, reports, service statistics, and budget requests.**

RATING	DESCRIPTOR
☐ 5	CF independently and consistently complies with administrative and regulatory policy requirements and does so in a timely and accurate manner. CF seeks supervisory guidance if needed.
☐ 4	
☐ 3	In most situations, CF independently complies with administrative and other regulatory policy requirements, although CF may need help with complex reports. Most information requested is provided in an accurate and timely manner. CF usually seeks supervisory guidance when needed.
☐ 2	
☐ 1	CF requires supervisory guidance to comply with administrative and other regulatory policy requirements. Information requested may be inaccurate and/or does not meet established time lines. CF does not seek supervisory guidance when needed.

13. **Uses local, state, national, and funding agency regulations to make decisions regarding service eligibility and, if applicable, third-party reimbursement.**

RATING	DESCRIPTOR
☐ 5	CF independently and accurately makes service eligibility decisions that are based on appropriate regulations and follows applicable mandates. CF seeks supervisory guidance if needed.
☐ 4	
☐ 3	In most situations, CF independently and accurately makes service eligibility decisions that are based on appropriate regulations and follow applicable mandates. CF usually seeks supervisory guidance when needed.
☐ 2	
☐ 1	CF requires supervisory guidance to make service eligibility decisions that are based on appropriate regulations. May not be able to follow applicable mandates even with direction. CF does not seek supervisory guidance when needed.
☐ NA	**NA** Not applicable. Skills not performed by CF at this facility.

Interaction Skills

*14. Demonstrates communication skills (including listening, speaking, nonverbal communication, and writing) that take into consideration the communication needs as well as the cultural values of the client, the family, caregivers, significant others, and other professionals.

RATING	DESCRIPTOR
☐ 5	CF independently presents information accurately, clearly, logically, and concisely. Oral communications, written reports, and letters are always appropriate for the needs of the audience. CF uses terminology and phrasing consistent with the semantic competency of the audience and includes accurate and complete information, listens carefully to clients and others, takes initiative in providing appropriate clarifications when needed, and demonstrates appropriate nonverbal communication style. CF seeks supervisory guidance if needed.
☐ 4	
☐ 3	CF usually presents information clearly, logically, and concisely. Oral communications, written reports, and letters are appropriate in most situations in that terminology and phrasing are consistent with the semantic competency of the audience. CF includes information that is accurate and/or complete. Listens to clients and others but may have difficulty providing appropriate clarification when needed. CF acknowledges the impact of own nonverbal communication style but may have difficulty demonstrating this consistently. CF usually seeks supervisory guidance when needed.

RATING	DESCRIPTOR
☐ 2	
☐ 1	CF does not present information clearly, logically, and concisely. Oral communication, written reports, and letters are inappropriate for the needs of the audience. CF uses terminology and phrasing inconsistent with the semantic competency of the audience and includes information that is inaccurate and/or incomplete. Does not listen carefully to clients and others and fails to provide appropriate clarification when needed. CF demonstrates inappropriate nonverbal communication style. CF does not seek supervisory guidance when needed.

*15. Identifies and refers clients for related services including audiological, educational, medical, psychological, social, and vocational, as appropriate.

RATING	DESCRIPTOR
☐ 5	CF consistently identifies the need for and makes appropriate client referrals. CF seeks supervisory guidance if needed.
☐ 4	
☐ 3	In most situations, CF identifies the need for client referrals but may need some assistance in locating specific referral sources. CF usually seeks supervisory guidance when needed.
☐ 2	
☐ 1	CF requires supervisory guidance to identify the need for client referrals and/or to make appropriate referrals. CF does not seek supervisory guidance when needed.

*16. Collaborates with other professionals in matters relevant to case management.

RATING	DESCRIPTOR
□ 5	CF consistently listens to input from others, makes appropriate decisions based on shared information, and initiates activities and contributes information that promotes mutual problem-solving. CF seeks supervisory guidance if needed.
□ 4	
□ 3	In most situations, CF listens carefully to input from others, makes appropriate decisions based on shared information, usually participates in activities and contributes information that promotes mutual problem-solving. CF usually seeks supervisory guidance when needed.
□ 2	
□ 1	CF requires supervisory guidance to effectively identify the need to consult or collaborate with other professionals in case management activities. Does not make decisions based on shared information and/or focus on mutual problem-solving activities. CF does not seek supervisory guidance when needed.

*17. Provides counseling and supportive guidance regarding the client's communication disorder to client, family, caregivers, and significant others.

RATING	DESCRIPTOR
☐ 5	CF listens, reflects, and explains information using terminology appropriate to the audience. CF monitors understanding by asking questions and encouraging interaction among all participants. Engages client/family in problem-solving activities. CF seeks supervisory guidance if needed.
☐ 4	
☐ 3	CF listens but may show some difficulty reflecting and/or explaining information using terminology appropriate to the audience. CF monitors understanding by asking questions but may have some difficulty encouraging interaction among all participants. CF attempts to engage client/family in problem-solving activities. CF usually seeks supervisory guidance when needed.
☐ 2	
☐ 1	CF does not listen, reflect, and/or explain information appropriately and does not use terminology appropriate to the audience. CF does not monitor understanding by asking questions and/or encouraging interaction among all participants. Does not engage client/family in problem-solving activities. CF does not seek supervisory guidance when needed

18. **Plans and implements educational programs for other professionals and the general public to facilitate acceptance and treatment of disabilities associated with communication disorders.**

RATING	DESCRIPTOR
□ 5	With consideration of the needs of the audience, CF independently and consistently provides clear and meaningful educational information to facilitate the acceptance and treatment of disabilities associated with communication disorders. CF seeks supervisory guidance if needed.
□ 4	
□ 3	In most situations, CF considers the needs of the audience and independently provides clear and meaningful educational information to facilitate the acceptance and treatment of disabilities associated with communication disorders. CF usually seeks supervisory guidance when needed.
□ 2	
□ 1	CF does not consider the needs of the audience and requires supervisory guidance to provide educational information that facilitates the acceptance and treatment of disabilities associated with communication disorders. CF does not seek supervisory guidance when needed.
□ NA	Not applicable. Skills not performed by CF at this facility.

APPENDIX C

Practicum Evaluation of Student Performance

Clinician:		Semester/Year:				
Circle One: Mid-semester Evaluation Final Evaluation		**Practicum Location:**				
	Rating Scale: 1 = Failing, 2 = Poor, 3 = Fair, 4 = Good, 5 = Excellent	**1**	**2**	**3**	**4**	**5**
1	**Clinicians Motivation:**					
	Is on time for sessions, conferences, practicum classes					
	Hands in lesson plans and other written material on time					
	Demonstrates effort and independence (e.g., creativity in developing therapy materials, extra time researching and integrating relevant information					
2	**Understanding of Goals and Procedures:**					
	Sets appropriate semester and session goals with clear rationales					
	Able to formulate behavioral goals					
	Understands levels of behavior (sequencing of goals)					
	Selects procedures appropriate to goals, patient's age and ability level					

continues

Rating Scale: 1 = Failing, 2 = Poor, 3 = Fair, 4 = Good, 5 = Excellent	1	2	3	4	5
3 Lesson Plan and Preparation:					
Write with correct grammar, spelling					
Uses clinical symbols and phonetic symbols properly					
Is developing adequate clinical statements of goals and procedures					
Is evaluating sessions with insight					
4 Application of Therapeutic Process:					
Gives adequate instruction					
Elicits appropriate responses in sufficient number					
Shapes responses accordingly					
Reinforces adequately					
Gives appropriate assignments					
5 Interaction with Patients:					
Listens					
Encourages patient communication					
Responds appropriately					
Shows flexibility					
6 Personal behavior:					
Dresses appropriately					
Uses acceptable voice, speech, and language					
7 Interaction with Supervisor:					
Listens					
Asks questions					
Incorporates suggestions					
8 Participates in Clinic					

	Comments: Any comment under a "4" requires a comment:
	Student Clinician:
	Supervisor's Signature:
	Grade Equivalent:

APPENDIX D

Supervisor Evaluation Form

Student's Name:			Semester/Year:		
Supervisor's Name:			Name of Site:		

Please put a "1" in the relevant box to rate each statement.	Disagree⟷Agree				
	1	2	3	4	5
1 I gained from the supervisor's knowledge and experience					
2 I received feedback in key areas important to my development					
3 My experience helped me develop a sharper focus on what is needed to grow professionally within the field					
4 I learned specific skills and knowledge that are relevant to <u>personal</u> growth					
5 I learned specific skills and knowledge that are relevant to <u>professional</u> growth					
6 I learned about the other areas and positions within the field					
7 I gained knowledge about the cultural and/or linguistic norms of a particular community					
8 My supervisor was a friendly ear with whom to share frustrations as well as successes					

continues

Please put a "1" in the relevant box to rate each statement.	Disagree⟷Agree				
	1	**2**	**3**	**4**	**5**
9	My supervisor discussed outcome/goal of the practicum with me					
10	My supervisor asked me about my background, goals, and aspirations					
11	My supervisor shared her/his expectations with me					
12	My advisor set realistic and focused goals for me					
13	My supervisor monitored my progress.					
14	My supervisor provided constructive feedback					
15	My supervisor encouraged me to take the lead in getting what I wanted from her/him					
16	I independently took the lead in getting what I wanted or needed from my supervisor					
17	My supervisor knows the organization (or field's) structure, policies, and processes					
18	My supervisor has a broad view and multiple working experiences					
19	My supervisor willingly shares knowledge and experiences					
20	My supervisor helps identify my strengths and developmental needs in a skill-set					
21	My supervisor generally tells, advises, instructs, suggests, and gives opinions					
22	My supervisor opened doors to opportunities within the field					

Please put a "1" in the relevant box to rate each statement.	Disagree⟷Agree				
	1	2	3	4	5
23 My supervisor made "an investment of faith" in my growth potential					
24 My supervisor was accessible and approachable					
25 My supervisor was generous with credit and praise					
26 My supervisor was encouraging after setbacks.					
27 My supervisor was a positive role model					
28 My supervisor practices what s/he preached					
29 My supervisor encouraged me to develop my own ideas by giving feedback that promotes a sense of independence, responsibility and self-confidence					
30 My supervisor provided feedback in the right environment					
31 I wanted honest input					
32 I tended to get defensive					
33 I listened carefully and asked for elaboration					
34 I expressed appreciation					
35 My supervisor was a coach not an accuser					
36 My supervisor was clear, concise and constructive					
37 My supervisor provided feedback in a timely fashion					

continues

Please put a "1" in the relevant box to rate each statement.	Disagree⟵⟶Agree				
	1	**2**	**3**	**4**	**5**
38	My supervisor provided academic input (i.e., information on population, history of school, printed material, access to files)					
39	I felt well-integrated within my site (i.e., routines, clinicians, school professionals, other personnel)					
40	I recommend my supervisor for training student clinicians					
41	I recommend my practicum site as a placement for student clinicians					
42	What did you learn?					
43	What could you have done better?					
44	What was your best experience as a supervisee? (i.e., What you vowed to repeat when you became a supervisor!)					
45	What was your worst experience as a supervisee? (i.e., What you vow to never do when you become a supervisor. What you vow you will do instead.)					
46	Please use this space to provide any other information you would like to disclose					

With acknowledgment to Teresa Signorelli for her contribution of the student and supervisor evaluation forms.

APPENDIX E

Supervisee Performance Assessment Instrument (SPAI)

The Supervisee Performance Assessment Instrument (SPAI) is a multi-faceted instrument that allows for self-assessment by the supervisee, collaboration between the supervisor and the supervisee, and/or supervisor assessment. The design of this instrument is to focus on the collaborative process between the supervisor and the supervisee through options of choosing both the evaluation criteria and the performance scale items. In developing this instrument as a collaboration tool, the authors decided to depart from many scales by introducing a large number of evaluation criteria and by using a nonhierarchical type of scaling. The rationale behind these two ideas is to provide the user with as much flexibility as possible in creating an evaluation tool that meets the needs of both the supervisor and supervisee. The format of the instrument allows the supervisor and supervisee to choose the specific areas for evaluation and tailor these to specific individuals or groups. The SPAI can be used by practicum and internship supervisors and as a tool for self-reflection.

Place the letter(s) of the instrument scale items chosen in the space preceding the criterion.

A. I have not been trained in using this skill.

B. I seldom use this skill.

C. I use this skill often.

D. This is a skill that does not fit my model/style.

E. I am comfortable using this skill.

F. I am uncomfortable using this skill.

G. I would like additional information and training on this skill.

Intervention Skills

_____ Listens to verbal and nonverbal communications

_____ Projects warmth, caring, and acceptance

_____ Communicates empathy and genuineness with clients

_____ Communicates effectively, using basic skills such as paraphrases, reflection questions, and summaries

_____ Establishes effective therapeutic relationships

_____ Observes in-session behavior (e.g., client language) and uses it to facilitate client/counselor relationship

_____ Uses silence as an effective intervention technique

_____ Times interventions to maximize effectiveness

_____ Attends to the relationship with clients

_____ Demonstrates readiness to explore charged areas

_____ Understands and uses resistance to assist clients

_____ Demonstrates effectiveness in making formal assessments

_____ Performs effective harm assessments

_____ Assists clients in goal-setting

_____ Helps clients build on their strengths

_____ Assists clients in assuming responsibility for their progress in therapy

_____ Assists clients in normalizing their behavior

_____ Understands how to help clients change their behavior

_____ Understands how to assist clients who are in crisis

_____ Demonstrates an ability to be concrete and specific

_____ Assists clients in identifying and exploring presenting problems

_____ Demonstrates the use of multiple approaches to treatment

_____ Works effectively with immediacy

_____ Exhibits control of the session

_____ Models effectively for clients

_____ Assists clients by partializing behavior

_____ Effectively uses reinforcement

_____ Rehearses new behaviors and skills with clients

_____ Effectively uses contracts and homework assignments

_____ Rehearses new behaviors and skills with clients

_____ Makes referrals when necessary

_____ Is knowledgeable about planned breaks, interruptions, and unplanned endings

_____ Is knowledgeable about termination:

    _____ Reviewing the treatment process

    _____ Giving and receiving feedback

    _____ Saying goodbye

Conceptualization Skills

____ Identifies relevant client themes and patterns

____ Assists clients in perceiving situations from different points of view

____ Assists clients in creating new perspectives

____ Uses client information to develop working hypotheses or hunches

____ Makes relevant observations about client behavior

____ Identifies and uses client discrepancies

____ Perceives underlying client issues

____ Uses client cultural background in assessment, diagnosis, and treatment

____ Encourages clients to hypothesize about their own behavior

____ Assists clients in developing relevant focus and direction

____ Evaluates the efficacy of interventions

____ Is knowledgeable about systems and their impact on the client

____ Accurately ascertains the reality of the client

____ Adapts theory and techniques to meet the client's reality

____ Grasps the complexity of issues involved with each client

____ Willing to reevaluate the conceptualization of the client

____ Diagnosis and treatment:

    ____ Identifies presenting symptoms and formulates DSM diagnoses

    ____ Formulates hypotheses based on client information

    ____ Develops appropriate strategies and interventions based on established theories and techniques

Professional Behavior

_____ Participates in continuing education activities such as supervision, courses, workshops, teaching, reading, writing

_____ Completes paperwork in a concise and timely manner

_____ Communicates written information clearly and effectively

_____ Communicates orally clearly and effectively

_____ Respects appointment times with clients and supervisors

_____ Possesses working knowledge of relevant professional literature

_____ Dresses appropriately

_____ Is aware and responsive to relevant ethical standards

    _____ Is knowledgeable about the profession's primary ethical standards

    _____ Effectively applies ethical standards to practice situation

    _____ Has begun to think ethically

    _____ Seeks consultation on complex ethical situations

_____ Is aware and responsive to relevant legal standards

_____ Makes a conscious effort to improve knowledge and skills

_____ Exhibits willingness to work on personal issues

_____ Exhibits respectful behavior toward clients and peers

_____ Demonstrates an awareness of personal influence and impact on clients

Supervision Skills for the Supervisee

_____ Initiates dialogue with the supervisor

_____ Arrives prepared at each supervision session

_____ Identifies questions, concerns, and issues relevant to current cases

_____ Creates professional development goals for supervision

_____ Shows interest in learning

_____ Understands and incorporates decisions

_____ Willing to take risks and identifying troublesome situations

_____ Seeks clarification of unfamiliar situations

_____ Accepts encouragement and constructive criticism

_____ Demonstrates concern and commitment to clients

_____ Actively participates in the supervisory process

From M. Fall & J. M. Sutton (2004). *Clinical supervision: A handbook for practitioners.* Boston: Allyn & Bacon. Reprinted with permission.

Knowledge and Skills Acquisition (KASA) Summary Form For Certification in Speech-Language Pathology

February 2009

Instructions for Use of the KASA Form

1. The CFCC encourages programs to use the KASA to demonstrate compliance with accreditation standards related to preparing students to meet ASHA certification requirements. However, programs may develop other documents to verify student's acquisition of knowledge and skills.

2. For academic programs and students wishing to use the KASA as a tracking document, indicate with a check mark in Column B whether each knowledge and skill was achieved. If a particular knowledge or skill was acquired through work completed in a specific course or courses, the title and number of the course(s) should be entered in Column C. If the knowledge or skills were acquired in clinical practicum, enter the title and number of the practicum in Column D. If the knowledge or skill was acquired through course work and/or clinical practicum, and/or lab or research activities, there should be entries in all of the applicable columns: C, D, and/or E.

3. Students and programs using the KASA are advised to keep a copy in a safe place, should they need to provide information at a later date (e.g., upon application for reinstatement).

4. CFCC encourages programs and students to periodically review the KASA (or other tracking documents developed by the program) to assist students in determining knowledge and skills already acquired and those yet to be attained.

Knowledge and Skills Acquisition (KASA) Summary Form For Certification in Speech-Language Pathology

The Kasa form is intended for use by the certification applicant during the graduate program to track the process by which the knowledge and skills specified in the 2005 Standards for the CCC are being acquired. Each student should review the KASA form at the beginning of graduate study, and update it at intervals throughout the graduate program and at the conclusion of the program.

The student, with input and monitoring of program faculty, must enter a check mark in column B as each of the knowledge and skills is acquired. It is expected that many entries will appear in the course work and the clinical practicum columns, with some entries, as appropriate, in the "Other" (lab, research, etc.) columns. Please enter the course or practicum number and title and description of other applicable activity.

KNOWLEDGE AREAS

A	B	C	D	E
			How achieved?	
Standards	Knowledge/ Skill Met? (check)	Course # and Title	Practicum Experiences # and Title	Other (e.g., labs, research) (Include description of activity)
Standard III-A. The applicant must demonstrate knowledge of the principles of:				
• Biological sciences				
• Physical sciences				
• Mathematics				
• Social/Behavioral sciences				

continues

KNOWLEDGE AREAS

A	B	C	D	E
			How achieved?	
Standards	**Knowledge/ Skill Met? (check)**	**Course # and Title**	**Practicum Experiences # and Title**	**Other (e.g., labs, research) (Include description of activity)**
Standard III-B. The applicant must demonstrate knowledge of basic human communication and swallowing processes, including their biological, neurological, acoustic, psychological, developmental, and linguistic and cultural bases				
• Basic Human Communication Processes				
• Biological				
• Neurological				
• Psychological				
• Developmental/Lifespan				
• Cultural				

242

Standard III-C. The applicant must demonstrate knowledge of the nature of speech, language, hearing, and communication disorders and differences and swallowing disorders, including their etiologies, characteristics, anatomic/physiologic, acoustic, psychological, developmental, and linguistic and cultural correlates. Specific knowledge must be demonstrated in the following areas:				
Articulation				
• Etiologies				
• Characteristics				
Fluency				
• Etiologies				
• Characteristics				

243

continues

KNOWLEDGE AREAS		How achieved?		
A Standards	**B** Knowledge/ Skill Met? (check)	**C** Course # and Title	**D** Practicum Experiences # and Title	**E** Other (e.g., labs, research) (Include description of activity)
Voice and resonance, including respiration and phonation				
• Etiologies				
• Characteristics				
Receptive and expressive language (phonology, morphology, syntax, semantics, and pragmatics) in speaking, listening, reading, writing, and manual modalities				
• Etiologies				
• Characteristics				
Hearing, including the impact on speech and language				
• Etiologies				
• Characteristics				

Swallowing (oral, pharyngeal, esophageal, and related functions, including oral function for feeding; orofacial myofunction)			
• Etiologies			
• Characteristics			
Cognitive aspects of communication (attention, memory, sequencing, problem-solving, executive functioning			
• Etiologies			
• Characteristics			
Social aspects of communication (challenging behavior, ineffective social skills, lack of communication opportunities)			
• Etiologies			
• Characteristics			

continues

KNOWLEDGE AREAS			How achieved?	
A	B	C	D	E
Standards	Knowledge/ Skill Met? (check)	Course # and Title	Practicum Experiences # and Title	Other (e.g., labs, research) (Include description of activity)
Communication modalities (including oral, manual, augmentative and alternative communication techniques, and assistive technologies)				
• Characteristics				
Standard III-D: The applicant must possess knowledge of the principles and methods of prevention, assessment, and intervention for people with communication and swallowing disorders, including consideration of anatomical/ physiological, psychological, developmental, and linguistic and cultural correlates of the disorders.				

246

Articulation			
• Prevention			
• Assessment			
• Intervention			
Fluency			
• Prevention			
• Assessment			
• Intervention			
Voice and Resonance			
• Prevention			
• Assessment			
• Intervention			
Receptive and Expressive Language			
• Prevention			
• Assessment			
• Intervention			

continues

KNOWLEDGE AREAS		How achieved?		
A	B	C	D	E
Standards	Knowledge/ Skill Met? (check)	Course # and Title	Practicum Experiences # and Title	Other (e.g., labs, research) (include description of activity)
Hearing, including the impact on speech and language				
• Prevention				
• Assessment				
• Intervention				
Swallowing (oral, pharyngeal, esophageal, and related functions, including oral function for feeding; orofacial myofunction)				
• Prevention				
• Assessment				
• Intervention				

Cognitive aspects of communication				
• Prevention				
• Assessment				
• Intervention				
Social aspects of communication				
• Prevention				
• Assessment				
• Intervention				
Communication Modalities				
• *(Prevention not applicable)*				
• Assessment				
• Intervention				

continues

KNOWLEDGE AREAS

A	B	C	D	E
			How achieved?	
Standards	Knowledge/ Skill Met? (check)	Course # and Title	Practicum Experiences # and Title	Other (e.g., labs, research) (Include description of activity)
Standard IV-G: The applicant for certification must complete a program of study that includes supervised clinical experiences sufficient in breadth and depth to achieve the following skills outcomes (in addition to clinical experiences, skills may be demonstrated through successful performance on academic course work and examinations, independent projects, or other appropriate alternative methods):				
1. Evaluation (must include all skill outcomes listed in a-g below for each of the 9 major areas except that prevention does not apply to communication modalities)				

a. Conduct screening and prevention procedures					
b. Collect case history information and integrate information from clients/patients, family, caregivers, teachers, relevant others, and other professionals					
c. Select and administer appropriate evaluation procedures, such as behavioral observations nonstandardized and standardized tests, and instrumental procedures					
d. Adapt evaluation procedures to meet client/patient needs					
e. Interpret, integrate, and synthesize all information to develop diagnoses and make appropriate recommendations for intervention					

continues

KNOWLEDGE AREAS		How achieved?		
A	B	C	D	E
Standards	Knowledge/ Skill Met? (check)	Course # and Title	Practicum Experiences # and Title	Other (e.g., labs, research) (Include description of activity)
f. **Complete administrative and reporting functions necessary to support evaluation**				
g. **Refer clients/patients for appropriate services**				
• Articulation				
• Fluency				
• Voice and resonance, including respiration and phonation				
• Receptive and expressive language (phonology, morphology, syntax, semantics, and pragmatics) in speaking, listening, reading, writing, and manual modalities				

• Hearing, including the impact on speech and language				
• Swallowing (oral, pharyngeal, esophageal, and related functions, including oral function for feeding; orofacial myofunction)				
• Cognitive aspects of communication (attention, memory, sequencing, problem-solving, executive functioning)				
• Social aspects of communication (including challenging behavior, ineffective social skills, lack of communication opportunities)				
• Communication modalities (including oral, manual, augmentative, and alternative communication techniques and assistive technologies)				

continues

KNOWLEDGE AREAS			How achieved?	
A	**B**	**C**	**D**	**E**
Standards	**Knowledge/ Skill Met? (check)**	**Course # and Title**	**Practicum Experiences # and Title**	**Other (e.g., labs, research) (Include description of activity)**
2. Intervention (must include all skill outcomes listed in a–g below for each of the 9 major areas)				
a. Develop setting-appropriate intervention plans with measurable and achievable goals that meet clients'/patients' needs. Collaborate with clients/patients and relevant others in the planning process				
b. Implement intervention plans (involve clients/ patients and relevant others in the intervention process)				

c. Select or develop and use appropriate materials and instrumentation for prevention and intervention				
d. Measure and evaluate clients'/patients' performance and progress				
e. Modify intervention plans, strategies, materials, or instrumentation as appropriate to meet the needs of clients/patients				
f. Complete administrative and reporting functions necessary to support intervention				
g. Identify and refer clients/patients for services as appropriate				
• Articulation				
• Fluency				

continues

KNOWLEDGE AREAS

A	B	C	D	E
	Knowledge/ Skill Met? (check)	**How achieved?**		
Standards	Knowledge/ Skill Met? (check)	Course # and Title	Practicum Experiences # and Title	Other (e.g., labs, research) (Include description of activity)
• Voice and resonance				
• Receptive and expressive language				
• Hearing, including the impact on speech and language				
• Swallowing				
• Cognitive aspects of communication				
• Social aspects of communication				
• Communication modalities				
3. Interaction and Personal Qualities				

a. Communicate effectively, recognizing the needs, values, preferred mode of communication, and cultural/linguistic background of the client/patient, family, caregivers, and relevant others.			
b. Collaborate with other professionals in case management.			
c. Provide counseling regarding communication and swallowing disorders to clients/patients, family, caregivers, and relevant others.			
d. Adhere to the ASHA Code of Ethics and behave professionally.			

APPENDIX G

ASHA Code of Ethics

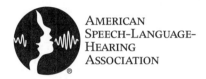

AMERICAN
SPEECH-LANGUAGE-
HEARING
ASSOCIATION

Preamble

The preservation of the highest standards of integrity and ethical principles is vital to the responsible discharge of obligations by speech-language pathologists, audiologists, and speech, language, and hearing scientists. This Code of Ethics sets forth the fundamental principles and rules considered essential to this purpose.

Every individual who is (a) a member of the American Speech-Language-Hearing Association, whether certified or not, (b) a nonmember holding the Certificate of Clinical Competence from the Association, (c) an applicant for membership or certification, or (d) a Clinical Fellow seeking to fulfill standards for certification shall abide by this Code of Ethics.

Any violation of the spirit and purpose of this Code shall be considered unethical. Failure to specify any particular responsibility or practice in this Code of Ethics shall not be construed as denial of the existence of such responsibilities or practices.

The fundamentals of ethical conduct are described by Principles of Ethics and by Rules of Ethics as they relate to the responsibility to persons served, the public, speech-language pathologists, audiologists, and speech, language, and hearing scientists, and to the conduct of research and scholarly activities.

Principles of Ethics, aspirational and inspirational in nature, form the underlying moral basis for the Code of Ethics. Individuals shall observe these principles as affirmative obligations under all conditions of professional activity.

Rules of Ethics are specific statements of minimally acceptable professional conduct or of prohibitions and are applicable to all individuals.

Principle of Ethics I

Individuals shall honor their responsibility to hold paramount the welfare of persons they serve professionally or who are participants in research and scholarly activities, and they shall treat animals involved in research in a humane manner.

Rules of Ethics

A. Individuals shall provide all services competently.

B. Individuals shall use every resource, including referral when appropriate, to ensure that high-quality service is provided.

C. Individuals shall not discriminate in the delivery of professional services or the conduct of research and scholarly activities on the basis of race or ethnicity, gender, gender identity/gender expression, age, religion, national origin, sexual orientation, or disability.

D. Individuals shall not misrepresent the credentials of assistants, technicians, support personnel, students, Clinical Fellows, or any others under their supervision, and they shall inform those they serve professionally of the name and professional credentials of persons providing services.

E. Individuals who hold the Certificate of Clinical Competence shall not delegate tasks that require the unique skills, knowledge, and judgment that are within the scope of their profession to assistants, technicians, support personnel, or any nonprofessionals over whom they have supervisory responsibility.

F. Individuals who hold the Certificate of Clinical Competence may delegate tasks related to provision of clinical services to assistants, technicians, support personnel, or any other persons only if those services are appropriately supervised, realizing that the responsibility for client welfare remains with the certified individual.

G. Individuals who hold the Certificate of Clinical Competence may delegate tasks related to provision of clinical services that require the unique skills, knowledge, and judgment that are within the scope of practice of their profession to students only if those services are appropriately supervised. The responsibility for client welfare remains with the certified individual.

H. Individuals shall fully inform the persons they serve of the nature and possible effects of services rendered and products dispensed, and they shall inform participants in research about the possible effects of their participation in research conducted.

I. Individuals shall evaluate the effectiveness of services rendered and of products dispensed, and they shall provide services or dispense products only when benefit can reasonably be expected.

J. Individuals shall not guarantee the results of any treatment or procedure, directly or by implication; however, they may make a reasonable statement of prognosis.

K. Individuals shall not provide clinical services solely by correspondence.

L. Individuals may practice by telecommunication (e.g., telehealth/e-health), where not prohibited by law.

M. Individuals shall adequately maintain and appropriately secure records of professional services rendered, research and scholarly activities conducted, and products dispensed, and they shall allow access to these records only when authorized or when required by law.

N. Individuals shall not reveal, without authorization, any professional or personal information about identified persons served professionally or identified participants involved in research and scholarly activities unless doing so is necessary to protect the welfare of the person or of the community or is otherwise required by law.

O. Individuals shall not charge for services not rendered, nor shall they misrepresent services rendered, products dispensed, or research and scholarly activities conducted.

P. Individuals shall enroll and include persons as participants in research or teaching demonstrations only if their participation is voluntary, without coercion, and with their informed consent.

Q. Individuals whose professional services are adversely affected by substance abuse or other health-related conditions shall seek professional assistance and, where appropriate, withdraw from the affected areas of practice.

R. Individuals shall not discontinue service to those they are serving without providing reasonable notice.

Principle of Ethics II

Individuals shall honor their responsibility to achieve and maintain the highest level of professional competence and performance.

Rules of Ethics

A. Individuals shall engage in the provision of clinical services only when they hold the appropriate Certificate of Clinical Competence or when they are in the certification process and are supervised by an individual who holds the appropriate Certificate of Clinical Competence.

B. Individuals shall engage in only those aspects of the professions that are within the scope of their professional practice and competence, considering their level of education, training, and experience.

C. Individuals shall engage in lifelong learning to maintain and enhance professional competence and performance.

D. Individuals shall not require or permit their professional staff to provide services or conduct research activities that exceed the staff member's competence, level of education, training, and experience.

E. Individuals shall ensure that all equipment used to provide services or to conduct research and scholarly activities is in proper working order and is properly calibrated.

Principle of Ethics III

Individuals shall honor their responsibility to the public by promoting public understanding of the professions, by supporting the development of services designed to fulfill the unmet needs of the public, and by providing accurate information in all communications involving any aspect of the professions, including the dissemination of research findings and scholarly activities, and the promotion, marketing, and advertising of products and services.

Rules of Ethics

A. Individuals shall not misrepresent their credentials, competence, education, training, experience, or scholarly or research contributions.

B. Individuals shall not participate in professional activities that constitute a conflict of interest.

C. Individuals shall refer those served professionally solely on the basis of the interest of those being referred and not on any personal interest, financial or otherwise.

D. Individuals shall not misrepresent research, diagnostic information, services rendered, results of services rendered, products dispensed, or the effects of products dispensed.

E. Individuals shall not defraud or engage in any scheme to defraud in connection with obtaining payment, reimbursement, or grants for services rendered, research conducted, or products dispensed.

F. Individuals' statements to the public shall provide accurate information about the nature and management of communication disorders, about the professions, about professional services, about products for sale, and about research and scholarly activities.

G. Individuals' statements to the public when advertising, announcing, and marketing their professional services; reporting research results; and promoting products shall adhere to professional standards and shall not contain misrepresentations.

Principle of Ethics IV

Individuals shall honor their responsibilities to the professions and their relationships with colleagues, students, and members of other professions and disciplines.

Rules of Ethics

A. Individuals shall uphold the dignity and autonomy of the professions, maintain harmonious interprofessional and intraprofessional relationships, and accept the professions' self-imposed standards.

B. Individuals shall prohibit anyone under their supervision from engaging in any practice that violates the Code of Ethics.

C. Individuals shall not engage in dishonesty, fraud, deceit, or misrepresentation.

D. Individuals shall not engage in any form of unlawful harassment, including sexual harassment or power abuse.

E. Individuals shall not engage in any other form of conduct that adversely reflects on the professions or on the individual's fitness to serve persons professionally.

F. Individuals shall not engage in sexual activities with clients, students, or research participants over whom they exercise professional authority or power.

G. Individuals shall assign credit only to those who have contributed to a publication, presentation, or product. Credit shall be assigned in proportion to the contribution and only with the contributor's consent.

H. Individuals shall reference the source when using other persons' ideas, research, presentations, or products in written, oral, or any other media presentation or summary.

I. Individuals' statements to colleagues about professional services, research results, and products shall adhere to prevailing professional standards and shall contain no misrepresentations.

J. Individuals shall not provide professional services without exercising independent professional judgment, regardless of referral source or prescription.

K. Individuals shall not discriminate in their relationships with colleagues, students, and members of other professions and disciplines on the basis of race or ethnicity, gender, gender identity/ gender expression, age, religion, national origin, sexual orientation, or disability.

L. Individuals shall not file or encourage others to file complaints that disregard or ignore facts that would disprove the allegation, nor should the Code of Ethics be used for personal reprisal, as a means of addressing personal animosity, or as a vehicle for retaliation.

M. Individuals who have reason to believe that the Code of Ethics has been violated shall inform the Board of Ethics.

N. Individuals shall comply fully with the policies of the Board of Ethics in its consideration and adjudication of complaints of violations of the Code of Ethics.

Reprinted with permission from American Speech-Language-Hearing Association. (2010). Code of Ethics [Ethics]. Available from www.asha.org/policy.

APPENDIX H

Mentoring Questionnaire

Mentoring is a developmental partnership through which one person shares knowledge, skills, information, and perspective to foster the personal and professional growth of someone else. As the interest in mentoring grows across many professions for the purposes of professional development for mentors and mentees, and as a way of ensuring the growth and vitality of the professions, we are interested in understanding the personal experience in mentorship. Because of your role in the profession, we believe that you can shed light on the meaning of mentoring and how it shapes professionals' lives. Please use the following questionnaire and brief rating scale as a guide to reflect on your own mentorship experiences as well as to examine your own beliefs about important issues pertaining to supervision and mentorship.

1. Background Summary of Interviewee:

   _____

   _____

   _____

   _____

   _____

   _____

2. A thumbnail sketch of the roles you have had as a professional.

_____

_____

_____

_____

_____

_____

Questions and Probes:

1. Did you have a mentor?

2. How did your pick your mentor? Why?

3. Conversely, did he or she or someone else select you to mentor?

4. How did your mentor help you?

5. Have you mentored students and/or professionals?

6. In what settings?

7. How did you do this?

   a. Probes: Listening, advising, providing opportunities: including your mentee in your work, introducing your mentee to others, etc.

8. What made your experiences successful?

9. What made your experiences unsuccessful?

10. How do you define mentoring with references to your experiences?

11. Do you think there is confusion among the terms/concepts of:

    a. Supervisor

    b. Role-model

    c. Mentor

12. Do cultural differences and/or gender differences affect the success of the process? If so, how?

On a scale of 1–5, please rate your opinion on the importance of mentorship to a successful career in speech-language pathology:

    1—Not important

    2—Somewhat important

    3—Moderately important

    4—Significantly important

    5—Exceptionally important

Contributed by Dr. Ann Jablon. Reprinted with permission.

APPENDIX I

Sample Enrollment Form Questions for ASHA S.T.E.P. Mentoring Program

Questions for Mentees	Questions for Mentors
Account Number	Account Number
First Name	First Name
Last Name	Last Name
Address	
City	
State	State
Country	
Zip Code	
Home Phone Number	Home Phone Number
Cell Phone Number	Cell Phone Number

continues

Questions for Mentees	Questions for Mentors
Account Number	Account Number
Would you accept text messages?	Would you accept text messages?
E-mail	E-mail
Area of Study	Area of Practice
Degree	Degree
Graduation Date	Years of Experience
University	
University Campus	
University Location	
What is your preference for being matched with a mentor from your university program?	What is your preference for being matched with a student from your university?
Clinical Age Population	Clinical Age Population You Work With
Employment Function	Employment Function
Employment Facility	Employment Facility
Specialty Areas	Specialty Areas

Questions for Mentees	Questions for Mentors
Account Number	Account Number
Spoken Languages	Spoken Languages
What are your career goals? (open-ended essay)	
How did you hear about the program?	How did you hear about the program?
Gender	Gender
Ethnicity	Ethnicity
Race	Race

Contributed by Andrea Moxley. Reprinted with permission.

APPENDIX J

Sample Year-End Survey for ASHA S.T.E.P. Mentoring Program

1. How likely are you to recommend this program to a student or colleague? Why or why not?

   ☐ Not at all likely   ☐ Not very likely   ☐ Pretty likely
   ☐ Very likely   ☐ I don't know

Questions Asked of Mentee Only

2. Please answer each of the following questions:

   ■ Did you write down goals for this program?

   ■ Did you review your program goals, written or unwritten, with your mentor?

   ■ Did the information and resources that your mentor provided help you achieve your goals?

   ■ Would you say that the relationship that you established with your mentor contributed to the success of your goals?

3. How successful do you feel you were at accomplishing the goals that you set for this program?

   ☐ Not at all successful   ☐ Not very successful
   ☐ Pretty successful   ☐ Very successful   ☐ I don't know

4. Have you ever applied for any of the following ASHA award programs? (Select all that apply.)

   ☐ Minority Student Leadership Program (MSLP)

   ☐ Research Mentoring Pair Travel Award

   ☐ Student Ethics Essay Award (SEEA)

   ☐ Students Preparing for Academic & Research Careers (SPARC) Award

   ☐ Student Research Travel Award

Questions Asked of Mentors Only

5. Have you ever participated in any of the following ASHA volunteer opportunities? (Select all that apply.)

   ☐ Peer Review

   ☐ ASHA Board, Council Committee

   ☐ ASHA Special Interest Division

   ☐ Expert review for grants and awards

   ☐ Contribute to the ASHA Leader

   ☐ Other (Fill in)

6. If no, why not?

7. Have you ever applied for any of the following ASHA award programs? (Select all that apply.)

   ☐ Advancing Academic-Research Careers (AARC) Award

   ☐ Audiology/Hearing Science Research Travel Award (ARTA)

   ☐ International Research Travel Award (IRTA)

   ☐ Research Mentoring-Pair Travel Award

☐ Clinical Practice Research Institute (CPRI)

☐ Lessons for Success

☐ Research Symposium Sponsored by NIDCD

☐ Grant Review and Reviewer Training Sponsored by the American Speech-Language-Hearing Foundation (ASHF) and ASHA's Research and Scientific Affairs Committee (RSAC)

☐ Projects on Multicultural Activities grant

Questions Asked of All Respondents

8. Which of the following resources did you use? (Select all that apply.)

   ☐ *Writing Mentoring Goals and Objectives* worksheet

   ☐ *The ASHA Gathering Place Mentoring Manual*

   ☐ Student section of ASHA Web site

   ☐ S.T.E.P. E-mails/newsletters

9. Which of the following social media channels do you use? (Select all that apply.)

   ☐ Facebook

   ☐ Twitter

   ☐ LinkedIn

   ☐ Other (Please specify)

10. Are you following ASHA S.T.E.P. Mentoring Program on Facebook? On Twitter?

11. What Facebook discussions would you participate in? Or Tweets?

12. What did you like most about the S.T.E.P. program?

13. What do you feel could be improved about the S.T.E.P. program?

14. Are there any additional E-mail and newsletter topics that you would find useful?

Contributed by Andrea Moxley. Reprinted with permission.

References

Abesamis, T. M. (2005). A guiding hand. *Advance, 15*(40), 10–11.

Abesamis, T. M. (2007). Mentoring students around the world. *The American Speech-Language and Hearing Association Leader Online.* Retrieved from http://www.asha.org/about/publications/leader-online/Letters Archive/ltr051018b

Aguilar, L. C. (2006). *Ouch! That stereotype hurts.* Flower Mound, TX: The Walk The Talk Company.

Allmark, P. (1995). A classical view of the theory-practice gap in nursing. *Journal of Advanced Nursing, 22*(1), 18–23.

American Speech-Language-Hearing Association. (n.d. [a]). *Exemplary practices in recruitment, retention and career transition of racial/ethnic minorities to communication science disorders.* Retrieved from http://www.asha.org/practice/multicultural/recruit/exemplarypractices.htm

American Speech-Language-Hearing Association. (n.d.[b]). *Writing mentoring goals and objectives.* Retrieved from http://www.asha.org/students/gatheringplace/step/goals.htm

American Speech-Language-Hearing Association. (1994). *Handbook of research education in communication sciences and disorders: A guide for program directors, research mentors, and prospective PhD students.* Rockville, MD: Research and Scientific Affairs Committee.

American Speech-Language-Hearing Association. (1996). Guidelines for the training, credentialing, use, and supervision of speech-language pathology assistants. *ASHA Task Force on Support Personnel, 37* (Suppl. 14), 21.

American Speech-Language-Hearing Association. (2003). *Knowledge and skills acquisition summary form for certification in speech-language pathology.* Retrieved from http://www.asha.org/uploadedFiles/KASA SummaryFormSLP.pdf

American Speech-Language-Hearing Association. (2004a). *Mentoring: The ASHA gathering place.* Retrieved from http://www.asha.org/students/gatheringplace/

American Speech-Language-Hearing Association. (2004b). *Report of the joint coordinating committee on evidence-based practice.* Retrieved from http://www.asha.org/uploadedFiles/members/ebp/JCCEBPRe port04.pdf

American Speech-Language-Hearing Association. (2004c). *Knowledge and skills needed by speech-language pathologists and audiologists to provide culturally and linguistically appropriate services* [Knowledge and skills]. Available from http://www.asha.org/policy/

American Speech-Language-Hearing Association. (2005). *Evidence-based practice in communication disorders* [Position statement]. Retrieved from http://www.asha.org/docs/html/PS2005-00221.html

American Speech-Language-Hearing Association. (2007a). *Responsibilities of individuals who mentor clinical fellows* [Issues in ethics]. Retrieved from http://www.asha.org/policy

American Speech-Language-Hearing Association. (2007b). *2006 S.T.E.P. program evaluation report.* Rockville, MD: Author.

American Speech-Language-Hearing Association. (2008a). *Clinical supervision in speech-language pathology* [Technical report]. Available from http://www.asha.org/policy

American Speech-Language-Hearing Association. (2008b). *Knowledge and skills needed by speech-language pathologists providing clinical supervision* [Knowledge and skills]. Available from http://www.asha.org/policy

American Speech-Language-Hearing Association. (2008c). *Your job . . . your career 2007. Summary report: Number and type of responses.* Rockville, MD: Author.

American Speech-Language-Hearing Association. (2008d). *2007 S.T.E.P. program evaluation report.* Rockville, MD: ASHA.

American Speech-Language-Hearing Association. (2009a). *Highlights and trends: ASHA counts for year end 2009.* Retrieved from http://www.asha.org/uploadedFiles/2009MemberCounts.pdf

American Speech-Language-Hearing Association. (2009b). *Knowledge and skills acquisition (KASA) summary form for certification in speech-language pathology.* Retrieved from http://www.asha.org/uploaded Files/certification/KASASummaryFormSLP.pdf

American Speech-Language-Hearing Association. (2009c). *2008 S.T.E.P. program evaluation report.* Rockville, MD: Author.

American Speech-Language-Hearing Association (2010a). *2009 S.T.E.P. program evaluation report.* Rockville, MD: Author.

American Speech-Language-Hearing Association. (2010b). *Certification.* Retrieved from http://www.asha.org/about/membership-certification/

American Speech-Language Hearing Association. (2010c). *Compendium of EBP guidelines and systematic reviews.* Retrieved from http://www.asha.org/members/ebp/compendium/

American Speech-Language-Hearing Association. (2010d). *Division 11, administration and supervision.* Retrieved from http://www.asha.org/members/divs/div_11.htm

American Speech-Language-Hearing Association. (2010e). *Information for clinical fellowship (CF) mentoring SLP's.* Retrieved from http://www.asha.org/certification/CFSupervisors.htm

American Speech-Language-Hearing Association. (2010f). *Mentorship in communication sciences and disorders.* Retrieved from http://www.asha.org/students/academic/doctoral/mentorship.htm

American-Speech-Language-Hearing Association. (2010g). *Code of ethics* [Ethics]. Available from http://www.asha.org/policy

American-Speech-Language-Hearing Association (2010h) *Frequently asked questions: Minority student leadership program.* Retrieved from http://www.asha.org/students/mslp.htm#7

Anderson, J. L. (1973). Supervision: The neglected component of the profession. In L. Turton (Ed.), *Proceedings of a workshop on supervision in speech pathology.* Ann Arbor, MI: University of Michigan.

Anderson, J. L. (1988). *The supervisory process in speech-language pathology and audiology.* Austin, TX: Pro-Ed.

Anzaldúa, G. (1987). *Borderlands/La frontera: The new mestiza.* San Francisco, CA: Aunt Lute Books.

Bandura, A. (1997). *Self-efficacy: The exercise of control.* New York, NY: Freeman.

Barrow, M., & Domingo, R. A. (1997). The effectiveness of training clinical supervisors in conducting the supervisory conference. *Clinical Supervisor, 16*(1), 55–78.

Battle, D. (2007, February 13). The power of passionate mentoring: Mentoring: The cycle of caring. *ASHA Leader,* 12.

Behrens, S. J. (2007). Case studies: When N of 1 is significant. *Field Notes, 3*(2), 14–15.

Behrens, S. J., & Carozza, L. (2007). *Emily and Dr. Haskins: Classroom expectations, pragmatics and clinical acumen.* Retrieved from http://www.sciencecases.org/emily/emily.asp

Behrens, S. J., & Jablon, A. D. (2008). Speaker perceptions of communicative effectiveness: Conversational analysis of student-teacher talk. *Journal of College Science Teaching, 37*(3), 40–44.

Behrens, S. J., Jablon, A. D., & Neeman, A. R. (2007). A linguistic examination of student-teacher talk: Implications for communication across dyads. *Research and Teaching in Developmental Education, 23*(2), 3–14.

Blake-Beard, S., Murrell, A., & Thomas, D. (2006). *Unfinished business: The impact of race on understanding mentoring relationships.* Retrieved from http://hbswk.hbs.edu/cgi-bin/print.

Boone, D., & Stech, E. (1970). The *development of clinical skills in speech pathology by audio tape and videotape self-confrontation, final report.* Washington, DC: Bureau of Education for the Handicapped (DHEW/OE).

Bordes, V., & Arredondo, P. (2005). Mentoring and first year Latina/o college students. *Journal of Hispanic Higher Education, 4*(2), 114–133.

Brommer, C., & Eisen, A. (2006). First: A model to increasing quality minority participation in the scenes from the undergraduate to graduate level. *Journal of Women in Sciences and Minorities, 12*, 35–46.

Burlington-Edison School District. (2010). Rubrics for enhancing professional practice: Speech-language pathologist. Retrieved from http://www.be.wednet.edu/StaffResources/Pathwise/Speech%20Lang%20Path%20Rubric.doc

Carozza, L. S. (2002). The need for mentorship in the minority professoriate. *Journal of Hispanic Higher Education, 1*(4), 351–356.

Castellanos, J., Gloria, A. M., & Kamimura, M. (2006). *The Latina/o pathway to the PhD: Abriendo caminos.* Sterling, VA: Stylus.

Chabon, S., Hale, S., & Wark, D. (2008). Triangulated ethics. *ASHA Leader, 13*(2), 26–27.

Clark, R., & Johnson, W. B. (2000). Mentor relationships in clinical doctoral training: Results of a national survey. *Teaching of Psychology, 27*(4), 262–268.

Clemente, C. L. (2006). *The relationship between perceived supervisory roles, styles, and working alliances, and students' self-efficacy in speech-language pathology practicum experiences* (Ph.D. dissertation, Touro University International). Retrieved June 2, 2010, from Dissertations & Theses: Full Text.

Clifford, J. R., Macy, M. G., Albi, L. D., Bricker, D. D., & Rahn, N. L. (2005). A model of clinical supervision for pre-service professionals in early intervention and early childhood special education. *Topics in Early Childhood Special Education, 25*(3), 167–176.

Cogan, M. (1973). *Clinical supervision*. Boston, MA: Houghton Mifflin.

Contreras, F., & Gandara, P. (2006). The Latina/o Ph.D. Pipeline: A case of historical and contemporary under-representation. In G. Castellano & M. Kamimura, *The Latina/o pathway to the Ph.D.* Sterling, VA: Stylus.

Crawford, H. (2007). Using evidence-based practice in supervision. In H. Roddam & J. Skeat, *Embedding evidence-based practice in speech and language therapy: International examples* (pp. 51–58). West Sussex, UK: John Wiley & Sons.

Crutcher, B. N. (2007). Mentoring across cultures. *Academe, 93*(4), 44–48.

Dollaghan, C. A. (2007). *The handbook for evidence-based practice in communication disorders*. Baltimore, MD: Paul H. Brookes.

Dowling, S. (1979). The teaching clinic: A supervisory alternative. *ASHA, 21*(9), 646–649.

Dowling, S. (1983). Teaching clinic conference participant interaction. *Journal of Communication Disorders, 16*(5), 385–397.

Dowling, S. (1987). Teaching clinic conferences: Perceptions of supervisor and peer behavior. *Journal of Communication Disorders, 20*(2), 119–128.

Elman, R. J. (2006). Evidence-based practice: What evidence is missing? *Aphasiology, 20*(2), 103–109.

Epstein, L. (2008). Clinical therapy data as learning process: The first year of clinical training and beyond. *Topics in Language Disorders, 28*(3), 274–285.

Fall, M., & Sutton, J. M. (2004). *Clinical supervision: A handbook for practitioners*. Auckland, NZ: Pearson Education New Zealand.

Ferguson, A. (2008). *Expert practice—A critical discourse*. San Diego, CA: Plural.

Ferguson, A. (2010). Appraisal in student–supervisor conferencing: A linguistic analysis. *International Journal of Language and Communication Disorders, 45*(2), 215–229.

Field, L., Korell-Chavez, S., & Domenech Rodríguez, M. M. (2010). No hay rosa sin espina: Conceptualizing Latina-Latina supervision from a multicultural developmental supervisory model. *Training and Education in Professional Psychology, 4*(1), 47–54.

Fitzgerald, M. T. (2009). Reflections on student perceptions of supervisory needs in clinical education. *Perspectives on Administration and Supervision, 19*, 96–106.

French, N. K. (1997). A case study of a speech-language pathologist's supervision of assistants in a school setting: Tracy's story. *Communication Disorders Quarterly*, *18*(1), 103-110.

Friedlander, M. L., & Ward, L. G. (1984). Development and validation of the supervisory styles inventory. *Journal of Counseling Psychology*, *31*, 541-557.

Friedman, T. (2008). *The world is flat 3.0: A brief history of the twenty first century*. New York, NY: Picador.

Fry, R. (2002). *Latinos on higher education: Many enroll, too few graduate*. Washington, DC: Pew Hispanic Center.

Geller, E., & Foley, G. M. (2009). Broadening the 'ports of entry' for speech-language pathologists: A relational and reflective model for clinical supervision. *American Journal of Speech-Language Pathology*, *18*(1), 22-41.

Gillam, R. B., Roussos, C. S., & Anderson, J. L. (1990). Facilitating changes in supervisees' clinical behaviors: An experimental investigation of supervisory effectiveness. *Journal of Speech and Hearing Disorders*, *55*(4), 729-739.

Gillam, S. L., & Gillam, R. R. (2008). Teaching graduate students to make evidence-based intervention decisions: Application of a seven-step process within an authentic learning context. *Topics in Language Disorders*, *28*(3), 212-228.

Glaser, A. J., & Donnelly, C. (1989). Data-based supervision methods for speech-language pathology. *Language, Speech, and Hearing Services in Schools*, *20*, 296-304.

Goldhammer, R. (1969). *Clinical supervision*. New York, NY: Holt, Rinehart, and Winston.

Goldstein, B. A. (2008). Integration of evidence-based practice into the university clinic. *Topics in Language Disorders*, *28*(3), 200-211.

Gooden, J. S., Leary, P. A., & Childress, R. B. (1994). Initiating minorities into the professoriate: One school's model. *Innovative Higher Education*, *18*(4), 243-253.

Grieco, E., & Cassidy, R. (2001). *Overview of race and Hispanic origin: Census 2000 Brief*. Retrieved from http://www.census.gov/population/www/cen2000/briefs/

Gunter, C. (n.d.). *Supervision and the professions: Resources for supervision*. Retrieved from http://www.asha.org/academic/teach-tools/supervision-resources.htm

The Hardiness Institute, Inc. (2001). *HardiSurveyIII-R Test*. Retrieved from http://www.hardinessinstitute.com/Research_FAQs.htm

Hew, K., & Knapczyk, D. (2007). Analysis of ill-structured problem solving, mentoring functions, and perceptions of practicum teachers and mentors toward online mentoring in a field-based practicum. *Instructional Science, 35*, 1–40.

Hidecker, M. C., Jones, R. S., Imig, D. R., & Villarruel, F. A. (2009). Using family paradigms to improve evidence-based practice. *American Journal of Speech-Language Pathology, 18*, 212–221.

Higgs, J., & McAllister, L. (2007). Educating clinical educators: Using a model of the experience of being a clinical educator. *Medical Teacher, 29*(2–3), e51–e57.

Hispanic Caucus. (2009). *The Hispanic caucus*. Retrieved from http://www.ashahispaniccaucus.com/ashaconvention

Ho, D. W. L., & Whitehill, T. (2009). Clinical supervision of speech-language pathology students: Comparison of two models of feedback. *International Journal of Speech-Language Pathology, 11*(3), 244–255.

Howard, F. (2008). Managing stress or enhancing well-being?: Positive psychology's contribution to clinical supervision. *Australian Psychologist, 43*(2),105–113.

Hudson, M. W. (2009). *A model for supervision and mentoring in speech-language pathology.* Paper presented at the Pennsylvania Speech-Language and Hearing Association and the Florida Association of Speech-Language Pathologists and Audiologists.

Hudson, M. W. (2010). Supervision: Supervision to mentoring: Practical considerations. *Perspectives on Administration and Supervision, 20*, 71–75.

International Mentoring Association. (2006). Resources for higher education mentoring.

Jacobi, M. (1991). Mentoring and undergraduate academic success: A literature review. *Journal of Educational Research, 61*(4), 505–532. Retrieved from http://www.mentoring-association.org/membersonly/HigherEd/ResUniv.html

Jarvis, P. (1987). *Adult learning in the social context.* New York, NY: Croom Helm.

Jarvis, P. (2000). The practitioner-researcher in nursing. *Nurse Education Today, 20*, 30–35.

Johnson, A. (2006). Higher education in CSD. *ASHA Leader, 11*(5), 24–25.

Johnson, S. (2002). *Who moved my cheese?* New York, NY: G. P. Putnam's Sons.

Johnson, W. B. (2007). Transformational supervision: When supervisors mentor. *Professional Psychology: Research and Practice, 38*(3), 259–267.

Justice, L. M., & Pence, K. (2007). *Parent-implemented interactive language intervention: Can it be used effectively? EBP Briefs: A scholarly forum for guiding evidence-based practices in speech-language pathology, 2*(1). Retrieved from http://www.speechandlanguage.com/ebp/pdfs/2-1-mar-2007.pdf

Kelly, T., Kingma, R. M., & Robinson, R. (2010). Building and supporting a multi-stream clinical evidence-based network. In H. Roddam & J. Skeat (Eds.), *Embedding evidence-based practice in speech and language therapy: International examples* (pp. 129–138). London, UK: Wiley-Blackwell.

Kirby, D., Morris, H., & Sullivan, D.L. (2006). *Clinical supervision: What was I thinking?!* Retrieved from: http://www.txsha.org/Convention/pdf/Morris,%20Holly-Clinical%20Supervision.pdf

Knowles, M. (1970). *The modern practice of adult education: Andragogy vs. pedagogy.* New York, NY: Cambridge Books.

Knowles, M. S., Holton III, E. F., & Swanson, R. A. (2005). *The adult learner* (6th ed.). Burlington, MA: Elsevier.

Koch, C. (2009). *Impact of supervisory feedback on the development of clinical expertise* (doctoral dissertation). Retrieved from http://p8080-marps.library.nova.edu.ezproxylocal.library.nova.edu/MARPs/mydefault.aspx

Kolb, A. Y., & Kolb, D. A. (2005). Learning styles and learning spaces: Enhancing experiential learning in higher education. *Academy of Management Learning and Education, 4*(2), 193–212.

Lambie, G. W., & Sias, S. M. (2009). An integrative psychological developmental model of supervision for professional school counselors-in-training. *Journal of Counseling and Development, 87*(3), 349–356.

Lee-Wilkerson, D., & Chabon, S. S. (2008). Reflections on a rubric used to facilitate accurate and informative assessment. *Administration and Supervision, 18*(2), 58–66.

Livingston, J. A. (1997). *Metacognition: An overview.* Retrieved from http://gse.buffalo.edu/fas/shuell/cep564/metacog.htm

Lopez, M. H. (2009, October 7). *Latinos and education: Explaining the attainment gap.* Washington, DC: Pew Hispanic Center.

Lubinski, R., & Frattali, C. (2000). *Professional issues in speech-language pathology and audiology.* San Diego, CA: Singular.

Lubinski, R., Golper, L. A. C., & Frattali, C. M. (2007). *Professional issues in speech-language pathology and audiology* (3rd ed.). Clifton Park, NY: Thomson Delmar Learning.

Maddi, S. R. (2005). Hardiness as the key to resilience under stress. *Psychology Review*, *11*, 20-23.

Manderson, D. (1997). FAQ: Initial questions about thesis supervision in saw. *Legal Education Review*, *8*(2), 121-139.

Martino, N., & Melcher, J. (2006). *Recruitment of minorities into the profession.* Poster presented at the American Speech, Language and Hearing Association Convention: Miami, FL.

Mawdsley, B. L., & Scudder, R. R. (1989). The integrative task-maturity model of supervision. *Language, Speech, and Hearing Services in Schools*, *20*, 305-319.

McAllister, L. (2005). Issues and innovations in clinical education. *Advances in Speech- Language Pathology*, *7*(3), 138-148.

McAllister, L., Higgs, J., & Smith, D. (2008). Facing and managing dilemmas as a clinical educator. *Higher Education Research and Development*, *27*(1), 1-13.

McCarthy, M. P. (2009). The clinical educator's companion: The Web-based ASHA scope of practice. *Perspectives on Administration and Supervision*, *19*(10-12), 64-70.

McCarthy, M. P. (2010). Outcomes: Promoting reflective practice using performance indicator questionnaires. *Perspectives on Administration and Supervision*, *20*, 64-70.

McCrea, E., & Brasseur, J. (2003). *The supervisory process in speech-language pathology and audiology.* Boston, MA: Allyn & Bacon.

McCready, V., & Raleigh, L. (2009). Creating a philosophy of supervision through personal perspective. *Perspectives on Administration and Supervision*, *19*, 87-95.

Meilijson, S., & Katzenberger, I. (2009). Reflections on reflections: Learning processes in speech and language pathology students' clinical education. *Perspectives on Administration and Supervision*, *16*, 62-71.

Merriam, S. B., Caffarella, R. S., & Baumgarten, L. M. (2007). *Learning in adulthood: A comprehensive guide* (3rd ed.). San Francisco, CA: Jossey-Bass.

Mok, C., Whitehill, T., & Dodd, B. (2008). Problem-based learning, critical thinking, and concept mapping in speech-language pathology education: A review. *International Journal of Speech-Language Pathology*, *10*(6), 438-448.

Morehouse, C. R., Rodgers, T. H., & Waguespack, G. M. (2006*) Professional ethics: Walk the line.* Presented at the American Speech-Language Hearing Association Conference, Miami, FL.

Moses, N., & Shapiro, D. A. (1996). A developmental conceptualization of clinical problem solving. *Journal of Communication Disorders, 29*(3), 199–221.

Mysall, M., Levett-Jones, T., & Lathlean, J. (2008). Mentorship in contemporary practice: The experiences of nursing students and practicing mentors. *Journal of Clinical Nursing, 17,* 1834–1842.

Nasim, A., & Talley, C. (2005). Race, gender, and the politics of pedagogy in psychology. *Essays from E-xcellence in Teaching, Vol. 4.* Retrieved from the Society for the Teaching of Psychology Web site: http://list.kennesaw.edu/archives/psychteacher.html

National Aphasia Association. (2006). *Aphasia bill of rights.* Retrieved from http://www.aphasia.org/

National Education Association. (2005). *Mentoring programs in higher education.* Retrieved from http://www2.nea.org/he/phms.html

National Mentoring Partnership. (2010). *Mentor.* Retrieved from http://www.mentoring.org

Newman, W. (2001). The ethical and legal aspects of clinical supervision. *Division 11 Newsletter, 11*(3), 18–22.

Newman, W. (2005). The basics of supervision. *ASHA Leader, 10*(10), 12–31.

Newman, W. (2008). *Clinical education and the professions.* Retrieved from http://www.asha.org/academic/teach-tools/supervision.htm

Newman, W., O'Connor Cabiale, L., & Victor, S. (2006). *Supervision boot camp.* [PowerPoint slides]. Retrieved from http://www.eshow2000.com/.../handouts/855_SC10Newman_Wren_057394_110206082251.ppt

O'Callaghan, A., McAllister, L., & Wilson, L. (2005). Barriers to accessing rural pediatric speech pathology services: Health care consumers' perspectives. *Australian Journal of Rural Health, 13*(3), 162–171.

O'Connor, L. (2006, March 9). *Supervision of clinical fellows: A mentoring process. SpeechPathology.com.* Recorded Course 2466. Retrieved from the e-Learning section on http://www.speechpathology.com

O'Connor, L. (2008). A look at supervision in the 21st century. *American Speech-Language and Hearing Association Leader, 13*(5), 14.

O'Connor, L. (2010) *The mentoring process: A learning focused approach SpeechPathology.com.* Self-Study Course 3854. Retrieved from the e-Learning section on http://www.speechpathology.com

Oratio, A. (1977). *Supervision in speech pathology: A handbook for supervisors and clinicians.* Baltimore, MD: University Park Press.

Ostergren, J. (2008). *Working alliance, supervisory styles/role, and satisfaction with supervision of speech-language pathologists during their first year of professional service.* (Ph.D. dissertation, Claremont Graduate University). Retrieved June 2, 2010, from Dissertations & Theses: Full Text.

Owen, C., & Solomon, L. (2006). The importance of interpersonal similarities in the teacher mentor/protege relationship. *Social Psychology of Education, 9*, 83–89.

Owen, C. J., Soloman, L. Z., Mallozzi, L. L., Kline, L. R., & Wareham, C. A. (2007a). *Mentoring: A potential solution to professional burnout.* Presented at the conference of the Society for Industrial and Organizational Psychology, New York, NY.

Owen, C. J., Soloman, L. Z., Mallozzi, L., Kline, L. R., & Wareham, C. A. (2007b). *Mentors: Feeling good by doing well.* Presented at the American Psychological Association Convention, San Francisco, CA.

Pappas, N., McLeod, S., McAllister, L., & McKinnon, D. (2008). Parental involvement in speech intervention: A national survey. *Clinical Linguistics and Phonetics, 22*(4–5), 335–344.

Pershey, M. G., & Reese, S. (2002). Consumer satisfaction with speech-language pathology services in university clinics: Implications for student supervision. *Clinical Supervisor, 21*(2), 185–205.

Phillips, K., & Sherman, A. F. (2009, November 9). *The "professional continuum" of supervision: From graduate to clinical fellow.* Speech-Pathology.com, Recorded Course 3594. Retrieved from the e-Learning section on http://www.speechpathology.com

Powell, T. (1987). A rating scale for measurement of attitudes toward clinical supervision. *SUPERvision, 11*, 31–34.

Rahim, M. A. (1989). Relationships of leader power to compliance and satisfaction with supervision: Evidence from a national sample of managers. *Journal of Management, 15*(4), 545–556.

Queens University Belfast. (2010). Excerpt from the NIPSWP practice learning handbook Sept 07: Appendix 14. Retrieved from http://www.qub.ac.uk/schools/media/Media,85517,en.doc

Quevedo, S. (2007, January 23). January is national mentoring month. *The ASHA Leader Online.* Retrieved from http://www.asha.org/Publications/leader/2007/070123/070123f.htm

Reber, A. S. (1989). Implicit learning and tacit knowledge. *Journal of Experimental Psychology, 118*(3), 219–235.

Riordan, R. J., & Kern, R. (1994). Shazam!!! You're a clinical supervisor. *Family Journal, 2*(3), 259–261.

Rivera- Goba,M.V. & Nieto, S. (2007). Mentoring Latina nurses: A multicultural perspective. *Journal of Latinos and Education, 6*(1), 35–53.

Robey, R. (2004). Levels of evidence. *ASHA Leader, 9*(7), 5.

Robey, R., & Dalebout, S. (1998). A tutorial in meta-analyses of clinical outcomes research. *Journal of Speech-Language and Hearing Research, 41*, 1227–1241.

Roddam, H., & Skeat, J. (2010). *Embedding evidence-based practice in speech and language therapy: International examples.* London, UK: Wiley-Blackwell.

Roman, S. M., & Carozza, L. S. (2007). *Representation of Hispanic and Latino professionals in communication sciences and disorders.* Presented at the National Association of Hispanic and Latino Studies Conference, Baton Rouge, LA.

Rowden, R. W. (2007). *Workplace learning: Principles and practice.* Malabar, FL: Krieger.

Sackett, D. L., Rosenberg, W. M. C., Muir Gray, J. A., Haynes, R. B., & Richardson, W. S. (1996). Evidence-based medicine: What it is and what it isn't. *British Medical Journal, 312*, 71–72.

Sanchez, B., & Reyes, D. (1999). Descriptive profile of the mentorship relationships of Latino adolescents. *Journal of Community Psychology, 27*(3), 299–302.

Santiago, D. A., & Brown, S. (2004). *Federal policy and Latinos in higher education.* Washington, DC: Pew Hispanic Center.

Santos, S. J., & Reigadas, E. T. (2002). Latinos in higher education: An evaluation of a university faculty mentoring program. *Journal of Hispanic Higher Education, 1*(1), 40–50.

Saras, L., & Post, D. (2004). Supervisory responses to critical teaching incidents during speech-language therapy. *Clinical Supervisor, 23*(1), 121–137.

Schmidt, P. (2003, November 28). Academe's Hispanic future. *The Chronicle of Higher Education.* Retrieved from http://chronicle.com/weekly/v50/i14/14a00801.htm

Schön, D. (1987.) *Educating the reflective practitioner.* San Francisco, CA: Jossey-Bass.

Seger, C. A. (1994). Implicit learning. *Psychological Bulletin, 115*(2), 163–196.

Shapiro, D. A., & Anderson, J. L. (1989): One measure of supervisory effectiveness in speech-language pathology and audiology. *Journal of Speech and Hearing Disorders, 54*, 549–557.

Shapiro, D. A., & Moses, N. (1989). Creative problem solving in public school supervision. *Language, Speech and Hearing Services in Schools, 20*, 320-332.

Shilpi, J. (1998). An investigation of supervisory style in speech pathology clinical education. *Clinical Supervisor, 17*(2), 141-155.

Shilpi, J., & McAllister, L. (1999). An investigation of supervisory style in speech pathology clinical education. *Clinical Supervisor, 17*(2), 141-155.

Simonsen, L., Luebeck, J., & Bice, L. (2009). The effectiveness of online paired mentoring for beginning science and mathematics teachers. *Journal of Distance Education, 23*, 51-68.

Skeat, J., & Perry, A. (2008). Exploring the implementation and use of outcome measurement in practice: A qualitative study. *International Journal of Language & Communication Disorders, 43*(2), 110-125.

Smith, R. (1989). Research and supervision in polytechnics. *Journal of Further and Higher Education, 13*(1), 76-83.

Staub, K. J. (2009). Facilitating supervisee cultural fluency for a multicultural society. *Perspectives on Administration and Supervision, 19*, 45-50.

Swail, W. C., Cabrera, A. F., Lee, C., & Williams, A. (2005). *Latino students and the educational pipeline, part III: Pathways to the bachelor's degree for Latino students.* Washington, DC: Educational Policy Institute.

Trautman, S. (2007). *Teach what you know: A leader's guide to knowledge transfer using peer mentoring.* Upper Saddle River, NJ: Prentice-Hall.

Turton, L. (1973). *Proceedings of a workshop on supervision in speech pathology.* Ann Arbor, MI: University of Michigan.

Vega, B. E. (Unpublished narrative). *Studying while brown: A critical identity awareness of a Latina doctoral student.* Columbia University, New York.

Victor, S. (2001). Developing a course in supervision at the graduate level. *American Speech-Language and Hearing Association Division 11, Perspectives on Administration and Supervision, 11*(1), 4-5.

Victor, S. (2010) Coordinator's column. *Perspectives on Administration and Supervision, 20*(3), 83-84.

Wagner, B. T., & Hess, C. W. (1997). Supervisees' perceptions of supervisors' social power in speech-language pathology. *American Journal of Speech-Language Pathology, 6*, 90-95.

Walsh, K., Nicholson, J., Keough, C., Pridham, R., Kramer, M., & Jeffrey, J. (2003). Development of a group model of clinical supervision to meet the needs of a community mental health nursing team. *International Journal of Nursing Practice, 9*(1), 33–39.

Weddington, G. (2006). The power of passionate mentoring: Mentoring students for professional success. *ASHA Leader, 11*(15), 16.

Wheatley, M. J. (2006). *Leadership and the new science: Discovering order in a chaotic world* (3rd ed.). San Francisco, CA: Berrett-Koehler.

Whitmire, K. A., & Eger, D. L. (2003). *Issue brief on personnel preparation and credentialing in speech-language pathology.* Gainesville, FL: University of Florida, Center on Personnel Studies in Special Education.

Whitmire, K. A., & Eger, D. L. (2004). Personnel preparation and credentialing in speech-language pathology. *Journal of Special Education Leadership, 17*(1), 26–32.

Williams, A. L. (1995). Modified teaching clinic: Peer group supervision in clinical training and professional development. *American Journal of Speech-Language Pathology, 4*(3), 29–38.

Winstanley, W., & White, E. (2003). Clinical supervision: Models, measures, and best practice. *Nurse Researcher, 10*(4), 7–38.

Worrall, L. E., & Bennett, S. (2001). Evidence-based practice: Barriers and facilitators for speech-language pathologists. *Journal of Medical Speech-Language Pathology, 9*(2), 11–16.

Zakowski, L., Seibert, C., & VanEyck, W. S. (2004). Evidence-based medicine: Answering questions of diagnosis. *Clinical Medicine and Research, 2*(1), 63–69.

Zanello, C. A. (1989). *A comparison of supervisory methods in the supervision of graduate students in speech-language pathology.* Retrieved June 2, 2010, from Dissertations & Theses: Full Text.

Zipoli, J., Richard P., & Kennedy, M. (2005). Evidence-based practice among speech-language pathologists: Attitudes, utilization, and barriers. *American Journal of Speech-Language Pathology, 14*(3), 208–220.

Zubizarreta, R., Campoy, F. I., & Ada, A. F. (2004). *Authors in the classroom: A transformative education process.* Boston, MA: Allyn & Bacon.

Additional Resources

Adelphi University. (2010). *Sixth annual international interdisciplinary conference on clinical supervision*. Retrieved from http://socialwork.adelphi.edu/clinicalsupervision/

Anderson, H. (2001). Clinical teaching and mentoring: Vital in the development of competent therapists. *International Journal of Language and Communication Disorders, 36*(1), 138–143.

Best, D., & Rose, M. (1996). *Quality supervision: Theory and practice for clinical supervisors*. London, UK: W. B. Saunders.

Brown, J. (2007). Why supervision matters in health care settings. *ASHA Leader, 12*(2), 30–31.

Brown, M. C., Davis, G., & McClendon, S. A. (1999). Mentoring graduate students of color: Myths, models and modes. *Peabody Journal of Education, 74*(2), 105–118.

Chang, M., & Vilardi, T. (2009). *Writing-based teaching: Essential practices and enduring questions*. Albany, NY: State University of New York Press.

Contemporary Issues in Communication Science and Disorders. (2006). Evidence-based practice, p. 33.

Cutcliffe, J. R., Hyrkas, K., & Fowler, J. (2010). *Routledge handbook of clinical supervision: Fundamental international themes*. New York, NY: Routledge.

Dowling, S., & Shank, K. (1981). A comparison of the effects of two supervisory styles: Conventional and teaching clinic in the training of speech and language pathologists. *Journal of Communication Disorders, 14*(1), 51–58.

Duchan, J. (2008). *Getting here: A short history of speech pathology in America*. Retrieved from http://www.acsu.buffalo.edu/~duchan/new_history/overview.html

Florida Department of State. (2010). *Supervision of speech-language pathology assistants and audiology assistants*. Retrieved from https://www.flrules.org/gateway/ruleno.asp?id=64B20-4.004

Gaffney, N. A. (1995). *A conversation about mentoring: Trends and models*. Washington, DC: Council of Graduate Schools.

Grimes, T. (2010). *Mentor: A memoir*. Portland, OR: Tin House Books.

Gurin, P., Dey, E. L., Hurtado, S., & Gurin, G. (2002). Diversity and higher education: Theory and impact on educational outcomes. *Harvard Educational Review, 72*(3), 1–21.

Heckman-Stone, C. (2003). Trainee preferences for feedback and evaluation in clinical supervision. *Clinical Supervisor, 22*(1), 21–33.

Higgs, J., & Edwards, H. (1994). *Educating the beginning practitioner*. Oxford, UK: Elsevier Butterworth-Heinemann.

Higgs, J., & Jones, M. (2000). *Clinical reasoning in the health professions*. Oxford, UK: Elsevier Butterworth-Heinemann.

Juarez, C. (1991). Recruiting minority students for academic careers: The role of graduate students and faculty mentors. *Political Science and Politics, 24*(3), 539–540.

Kilminster, S. M., & Jolly, B. C. (2000). Effective supervision in clinical practice settings: A literature review. *Medical Education, 34*, 827–840.

King's College London. (2010). *Supervisory good practice*. Retrieved from http://www.kcl.ac.uk/content/1/c6/02/15/72/SupervisoryGoodPractice.doc

Kirby, D., Morris, M., & Sullivan, D. (2006). *Clinical supervision: What was I thinking?!* [PowerPoint slides]. Retrieved from http://www.txsha.org

Lai, B. S., & Ellison, W. D. (2007). Finding the right mentor: Gaining admission to and succeeding in graduate school: *Eye on Psi Chi, 11*(4), 16–19.

Lee, C., & Schmaman, F. (1987). Self-efficacy as a predictor of clinical skills among speech-pathology students. *Higher Education, 16*(4), 407–416.

Malone, R. (1999). *The first 75 years: An oral history of the American-Speech-Language-Hearing Association*. Washington, DC: American Speech-Language and Hearing Association.

Manathunga, C. (2007). Supervision as mentoring: The role of power and boundary crossing. *Studies in Continuing Education, 29*(2), 207–221.

McCrea, E. S., & Brasseur, J. A. (2003). *The supervisory process in speech-language pathology and audiology*. Upper Saddle River, NJ: Allyn & Bacon.

Mercaitis, P. (1988). Perceived utility of a self-evaluation procedure by students in speech-language pathology. *Clinical Supervisor, 6*(1), 21–32.

Moore, C. (2007). Mentoring moments. *ASHA Leader, 12*(1), 16–17.

Morehouse, C. R., Rodgers, T. H., & Waguespack, G. M. (2006, November 16). *Professional ethics: Walk the line.* Presentation at the American Speech-Language-Hearing Association: Miami, FL.

NSW Institute of Rural Clinical Services and Teaching. (2008). *A report: Clinical supervision for allied health professionals in rural NSW.* Retrieved from http://www.ircst.health.nsw.gov.au/_data/assets/pdf_file/0004/67936/Rural_NSW_Allied_Health_Clinical_Supervision_Paper_Final.pdf

Oliva, M. (2002). Access to doctoral study for Hispanic students: The pragmatics of race in (recent) Texas history and policy. *Journal of Hispanic Higher Education, 1*(2), 158–173.

Omi, M., & Winant, H. (1994). *Racial formation in the United States* (2nd ed.). New York, NY: Routledge.

Penn State University. (2010). *The mentor: An academic advising journal.*

Reilly, S., Douglas, J., & Oates J. (2004). *Evidence-based practice in speech pathology.* London, UK: Whurr.

Rosa-Lugo, L. I., Rivera, E. A., & McKeown, S. W. (1998). Meeting the critical shortage of speech-language pathologists to serve the public schools. *Language, Speech, and Hearing Services in Schools, 29,* 232–242.

Rose, M., & Best, D. (2005). *Transforming practice through clinical education, professional supervision, and mentoring.* London, UK: Elsevier.

Sauchey, B., & Reyes, D. (1999). Descriptive profile of the mentorship relationships of Latino adolescents. *Journal of Community Psychology, 27*(3), 299–302.

Sciavetti, N., & Metz, D. E. (2006). *Evaluating research in communicative disorders* (5th ed.). Boston, MA: Pearson Allyn and Bacon.

Shapiro, D. A., Ogletree, B. T., & Brotherton, W. D. (2002). Graduate students with marginal abilities in communication sciences and disorders: Prevalence, profiles, and solutions. *Journal of Communication Disorders, 35,* 421–451.

Sleight, C. C. (1990). Off-campus supervision self-evaluation. *Clinical Supervisor, 8*(1), 163–174.

Smith, K. (1989). The supervisory process: An introduction. *Language, Speech and Hearing Services in Schools, 20,* 269–273.

SpeechPathology.com

StateUniversity.com. (2010). *Supervision of instruction: The history of supervision, roles and responsibilities of supervisors, issues, trends, and controversies.* Retrieved from http://education.stateuniversity.com/pages/2472/Supervision-Instruction.html

SupervisionResource.com. (2005). *Supervision resource*. Retrieved from http://supervisionresource.com/

Taylor, C. L. (1996). *Considering student's reflections on their practice as an aspect of professional competence*. Proceedings from the Higher Education Research and Development Society of Australia Conference: Perth, Western Australia. Retrieved from http://www.herdsa.org.au/confs/1996/taylorcl2.html

Turner-Muecke, L. A. (1986). Reflection-in-action: Case study of a clinical supervisor. *Journal of Supervision, 2*(1), 40–49.

Wilding, C., Marais-Strydom, E., & Teo, N. (2003). MentorLink: Empowering occupational therapists through mentoring. *Australian Occupational Therapy Journal, 50*(4), 259–261.

Wyre Forest NHS. (2005). *Clinical supervision: Policy for the clinical supervision of nurses and allied health professionals (AHP's) in the provider services*. Retrieved from www.worcestershirehealth.nhs.uk/.../policies.../Clinical/150607ClinicalSupervisionPolicy.pdf

Index